The Pharmacy Student

Companion

Notice

The authors and the publisher have made every effort to ensure the accuracy and completeness of the information presented in this book. However, the authors and the publisher cannot be held responsible for the continued currency of the information, any inadvertent errors or omissions, or the application of this information. Therefore, the authors and the publisher shall have no liability to any person or entity with regard to claims, loss, or damage caused, or alleged to be caused, directly or indirectly, by the use of information contained herein.

The Pharmacy Student Companion:

Your Road Map to Pharmacy Education and Careers

Daniel H. Albrant, Pharm.D.
Linda R. Harteker

American Pharmaceutical Association
Washington, D.C.

Managing Editor: Julian I. Graubart
Graphic Designer: Christopher K. Baker
Art and Production Director: Mary Jane Hickey
Proofreaders: Roseann Neatrour, Susan C. Kendall

Library of Congress Catalog Card Number: 97-070173
ISBN 0-917330-84-6

© 1997 by American Pharmaceutical Association
All rights reserved
Published by the American Pharmaceutical Association,
2215 Constitution Avenue, N.W., Washinton, DC 20037-2985

No part of this book may be reproduced, stored in a retrieval system, or transmitted in any form or by any means, electronic, mechanical, photocopying, recording, or otherwise without written permission from the publisher.

Printed in the United States of America

How to Order This Book
By phone: 800-878-0729 (802-862-0095 from outside the United States).
VISA®, MasterCard®, and American Express® cards accepted.

Contents

List of Appendixes	vii
Foreword	viii
Acknowledgments	ix
Contributors	x

Chapter 1: Pharmacy Practice Today — 1
- Introduction — 1
- Pharmaceutical Care and Disease State Management — 6
- Pharmacist Profiles — 7
- Pharmacy ABC's — 17
- Will There Be a Job for Me in the Year 2002? In 2022? — 18

Chapter 2: Is Pharmacy the Career for You? — 21
- Introduction — 21
- How to Start — 22
- Pathways to Pharmacy — 22
- Which Degree Is Right for Me? — 22
- Admission Requirements — 23
- Choosing a Pharmacy School — 24
- Additional Resources — 24

Chapter 3: Pharmacy School: What You Can Expect — 29
- Introduction — 29
- The Pharmacy Curriculum — 30
- Graduate Programs in Pharmacy — 31
- Print Resources — 33
- Internet Addresses — 34

Chapter 4: Involvement in the National Professional Society of Pharmacists — 43
- Introduction — 43
- History of APhA-ASP — 44
- Governing Structure — 44
- Membership in APhA-ASP — 45
- Member Benefits — 45
- APhA-ASP Activities — 47

Chapter 5: The World of Pharmacy Organizations — 51
- Introduction — 51
- State APhA Associations — 51
- Organizations with Student Membership Categories — 52
- Organizations with Institutional Members — 54
- Other Pharmaceutical Organizations — 55
- Internet Addresses of Pharmacy and Other Health Organizations — 55

Chapter 6: Continuing Your Education: Residencies and Fellowships, *Linda K. Ohri* — 61
- Introduction — 61

Residency and Fellowship Programs	61	
Accreditation of Residency and Fellowship Programs	62	
ASHP Resident Matching Program	63	
Characteristics of Residency and Fellowship Programs	63	
Elements of Residency and Fellowship Training	64	
Benefits of Residency and Fellowship Training	65	
Preparing for a Residency or Fellowship	65	
How to Learn about Residencies and Fellowships	66	
RESFILE: Simplifying the Search	66	
Resources	67	

Chapter 7: Getting Your License — 95

- Introduction — 95
- State Boards of Pharmacy — 95
- Getting Licensed — 96
- Relicensure — 96
- Score and Licensure Transfer — 97
- "Oath of a Pharmacist" — 97
- Information for Foreign Pharmacy Graduates — 98
- NABP Resources — 100

Chapter 8: Landing Your First Position — 115

- Introduction — 115
- Job versus Career: What's the Difference? — 116
- Taking the First Steps in Your Career — 116
- Fine-Tune Your Search — 117
- Sources of Career Information — 118
- Networking — 119
- Applying for a Position: Cover Letters, Résumés, and Curricula Vitae — 120
- The Employment Interview — 121
- Making Your Decision — 123
- Print Resources — 123
- Other Resources — 124

Appendixes

A. U.S. schools and colleges of pharmacy 25

B. Scholarships, loans, awards, grants, internships, and research experiences 37

C. U.S. graduate programs in pharmacy, 1996-97 41

D. State pharmacy associations 57

E. RESFILE 97 residencies 69

F. RESFILE 97 fellowships 87

G. Planning time line for residencies and fellowships 91

H. Sample RESFILE program record 93

I. Sample inquiry letter generated by RESFILE 93

J. State boards of pharmacy 102

K. State licensure examination requirements 106

L. State internship requirements 107

M. State continuing-education requirements 110

N. State licensure transfer requirements 113

O. Sample cover letter to employer 126

P. Sample résumé 126

Q. Sample curriculum vitae 127

Foreword

Welcome to *The Pharmacy Student Companion*—the most important and useful book you may ever own.

If you are thinking about a career in pharmacy, you have chosen to explore the nation's most trusted health profession. *The Pharmacy Student Companion* will help you begin this exploration.

The *Companion* will also be invaluable to those who have already made a commitment to the profession. Whether you are a prepharmacy student, pharmacy student, guidance counselor, student adviser, faculty member, or practitioner, this resource can simplify your life.

The Pharmacy Student Companion is published by the American Pharmaceutical Association–Academy of Students of Pharmacy (APhA-ASP). With more than 50,000 members, APhA is the largest national professional society of pharmacists in the United States. APhA-ASP is the student section of the APhA. We have more than 18,000 members and maintain chapters at every school or college of pharmacy in the country. APhA-ASP members are the future of the profession of pharmacy. We are committed to becoming innovative practitioners and to providing and promoting patient-focused pharmaceutical care.

The *Companion* begins with information that will be of interest primarily to prepharmacy students or high school students. It continues with information about pharmacy school, the pharmacy curriculum, residencies and fellowships, postgraduate work, and licensure. Also featured are interviews with several contemporary pharmacists. Their experience will enable you to appreciate the scope of practice today. The book ends with information that will help you land your first pharmacist position. We've also included information on professional pharmacy organizations, the meaning of professionalism, and tips on how to market your skills. Most chapters end with a list of resources, including Internet addresses, that will be helpful to students and newly licensed pharmacists. No other document on pharmacy education and careers is this comprehensive!

Like thousands of other pharmacy students, I wish that this book had been available when I began my education. I encourage you to use it as your springboard to a great career. Pharmacy is a rapidly evolving profession, and the knowledge you gain in the classroom is only part of what you'll need to know. *The Pharmacy Student Companion* can enhance your education and will equip you to bring about a revolution in the profession of pharmacy.

I wish you all the best as you pursue your dream.

Your Colleague,

Joshua S. Benner
President, APhA–ASP

P.S. Because this is the first edition of *The Pharmacy Student Companion* and we plan to update it regularly, we're especially interested in your feedback. What sections do you find most helpful? Where could we improve? Please send your comments to Julian Graubart, Director, Books and Electronic Products Department, at APhA (1-800-237-APhA, ext. 7561 or jig@mail.aphanet.org).

Acknowledgments

The American Pharmaceutical Association (APhA) and the authors gratefully acknowledge the contributions of the following organizations and individuals whose support and efforts made possible the publication of *The Pharmacy Student Companion*.

The book, developed by APhA-ASP, was supported by an unrestricted educational grant from Merck U.S. Human Health Division. We extend special thanks to David G. Miller, Director of Pharmacy Affairs, for his vision and encouragement in producing this reference.

Two national organizations generously provided a wealth of information found in the book: American Association of Colleges of Pharmacy (AACP) and National Association of Boards of Pharmacy (NABP). We thank our primary contacts—Mark D. Boesen, Manager, Government and Student Affairs for AACP, and Janice Teplitz, Assistant Executive Director of NABP.

Linda K. Ohri, Assistant Professor of Pharmacy Practice, Creighton University School of Pharmacy and Allied Health Professions, generously permitted APhA to include a print version of RESFILE, a comprehensive database of pharmacy residency and fellowship programs. Dr. Ohri also wrote Chapter 6, Continuing Your Education: Residencies and Fellowships.

Tim Dey, the APhA-ASP Summer Intern in 1996, developed the grant proposal to publish this book, which included the preliminary content outline. The project was a high priority of the APhA-ASP Executive Committee: President Josh Benner (Drake University), President-elect Jessika Stewart (University of Kentucky), Speaker of the APhA-ASP House of Delegates Trey Gardner (University of Arkansas), and Members-at-Large Marci Catalano (Duquesne University) and Tim Dey (Philadelphia College of Pharmacy and Science).

S. Bruce Benson, Associate Director for Professional Relations, University of Minnesota College of Pharmacy, offered author Dan Albrant some helpful perspective during the planning stage on the shape the book should take. And 10 pharmacy students, whose observations appear in the book, donated their time to participate in a focus group with Dr. Albrant: Todd Addington (Shenandoah University), Jim Brown and Tim Dey (Philadelphia College of Pharmacy and Science), Marci Catalano and Amy Daugherty (Duquesne University), Jim Masterson (University of Pittsburgh), Melissa Parrish and Amy Whitaker (Medical College of Virginia), Charlotte Puglia (Wilkes University), and Darrell Willis (West Virginia University).

Thanks are extended as well to those pharmacists who granted interviews for the book's practitioner profiles: Timothy W. Ames, David Angaran, Dennis Cada, Donald A. Dee, Michael J. Groh, Grace Hayes, Brian J. Isetts, Anna Kowblansky, Michael Manolakis, Phyllis Moret, John Parisi, Leo J. Sioris, Greg Susla, Donna Walker-Pulido, and Lynn F. Williams.

Finally, for their determination to provide valuable resources that instill professionalism in America's pharmacy students, thanks to APhA staff members Jann B. Hinkle, Director of Student Affairs, and Charles M. Dragovich, Associate Director of Student Affairs.

Contributors

Daniel H. Albrant, Pharm.D., is President of Pharmacy Dynamics, Arlington, Virginia, a firm that helps clients solve medication-use problems. Previous positions include Clinical Coordinator, Critical Care and Transplantation, Department of Pharmacy Services, Fairfax Hospital, Falls Church, Virginia, and Affiliate Assistant Professor of Pharmacy Practice, Auburn University School of Pharmacy. He has published a number of professional papers, including the chapter "Effective Protocol Implementation Guided by TQM and CQI Principles" in the *APhA Guide to Drug Treatment Protocols: A Resource for Creating and Using Disease-Specific Pathways.*

Linda R. Harteker has been a health writer and editor in Washington, D.C., for more than 20 years and has worked on many APhA publications in recent years. She was Director of Public Information for the American Society of Health-System Pharmacists from 1984 to 1988.

Chapter 1
Pharmacy Practice Today

Introduction

What is pharmacy? It's the nation's third largest health profession. Today, there are approximately 170,000 licensed pharmacists in the United States.

Where do pharmacists work? The single greatest number—some 43,000—work in community pharmacies; however, pharmacists work in all areas of health care and medical research. They are employed in hospitals, nursing homes, home health care companies, managed care organizations, clinics, and physicians' offices. They hold both staff and management positions. Many pharmacists work for federal agencies such as the Food and Drug Administration and the National Institutes of Health, as well as for the U.S. armed forces and Department of Veterans Affairs. They are faculty members at colleges and universities. They do research in the pharmaceutical industry. Increasing numbers of pharmacists have dual degrees in law, computer technology, business administration, or other areas.

Tables 1 and 2 provide current information on the total number of licensed pharmacists and pharmacies in the United States today.

All pharmacists, regardless of practice setting or experience, share a single goal: to make sure that each of their patients uses medications as safely and effectively as possible.

This chapter introduces you to pharmacy—a fascinating, challenging, and promising career. It begins with an introduction to two exciting concepts in pharmacy today: pharmaceutical care and disease state management. Next come several interviews with con-

Table 1

Pharmacists - Number Licensed, Where They Practice* (July 1, 1995 - June 30, 1996)

| State | Total Licensed by State | Pharmacists with In-State Addresses | Total in Practice |||||
			Ambulatory/ Community Pharmacy	Hospital Pharmacy	Manufacturing/ Wholesale	Teaching/ Government	Other Capacities
Alabama	5,378	4,200	2,763	1,373	53	80	1,109
Alaska	443	314					
Arizona	5,200	3,200	1,820	550	30	220	330
Arkansas	3,039	2,242	894	551	15	44	49
California B	28,223	20,609					
Colorado	5,100 D	3,852					
Connecticut	4,085	2,760					
Delaware	922	471					
District of Columbia	1,350						
Florida	19,556	12,433					
Georgia	9,019						
Hawaii	1,253	730					
Idaho	1,366	801					
Illinois	11,792	9,105					
Indiana	6,591	4,636					
Iowa	4,697	2,634	1,458 F	508 F	16 F	63 F	235 F
Kansas	3,270	2,192					
Kentucky	4,670	3,800 D					
Louisiana	5,487	4,106	2,481	1,058	45	74	448
Maine	1,278						
Maryland	9,461	5,906	2,771	1,323	129	522	
Massachusetts	9,283						
Michigan	9,882	7,662					
Minnesota	5,109	3,834	3,250	1,323	148	262	126
Mississippi	3,215	2,319					
Missouri	6,102	4,057	2,005	987	65	2	421

Table 1 (cont.)

State	Total Licensed by State	Pharmacists with In-State Addresses	Total in Practice Ambulatory/ Community Pharmacy	Hospital Pharmacy	Manufacturing/ Wholesale	Teaching/ Government	Other Capacities
Montana	1,295	787			209		
Nebraska	2,332	1,542					
Nevada	6,353	1,098					
New Hampshire	1,623	799	546	176			
New Jersey	13,000 D						
New Mexico	1,997	1,251					
New York	18,042	14,804					
North Carolina	7,897	6,269	3,351	1,297	101	62	677 M
North Dakota	1,996	658	482	116	10	30	20
Ohio	12,831	9,537	4,907	2,014	107	88	1,115
Oklahoma	4,245	2,952 D					
Oregon	3,606	2,406					
Pennsylvania	15,919	12,192					
Puerto Rico	2,217	1,917	1,739	259	115	89	15
Rhode Island	1,700	895					
South Carolina	4,969	3,291	1,977	724	28	96	103
South Dakota	1,445	754	460	189	15	35	55
Tennessee	6,433	4,933	3,790	2,415			
Texas O	18,080	14,158	8,089	3,425	146	240	2,258
Utah	2,187				33	3	
Vermont	750	359					
Virginia	7,321	5,043					
Washington	5,779	4,433					
West Virginia	2,740	1,558					
Wisconsin	5,537	4,121					
Wyoming	1,024	433	317	55	0	9	2
Totals	317,089	198,053	43,100	18,343	1,265	1,919	6,963

* Information provided directly from the state boards of pharmacy. Blanks indicate that information is not available.
Reprinted with permission from the 1996-97 National Association of Boards of Pharmacy *Survey of Pharmacy Law.*

Table 2

Pharmacies - Number of Pharmacies Licensed* (July 1, 1995 - June 30, 1996)

State	Total Pharmacies	Hospital/ Institutional Pharmacies	Independent Community Pharmacies	Nonindependent Community Pharmacies (Four or More)	Out-of-State or Nonresident Pharmacies
Alabama	1,622	187	694	572	169
Alaska	107	13	94 A		69
Arizona	799	71	105	623	0
Arkansas	726	154	614	112	86
California C	5,849	662			118
Colorado	750				0
Connecticut	664	58	305	359	0
Delaware	138	13	25	113	95
District of Columbia	150	15	135	75	0
Florida	5,501	1,779	3,409 A	A	190
Georgia	2,312	220			
Hawaii	197				56
Idaho	451	56	224 A, E		109
Illinois	2,722	334	2,303	A	83
Indiana	1,391	181			
Iowa	1,059	132	789 A	A	127
Kansas	758				135
Kentucky	1,325	127	502	546	150
Louisiana	1,765 G	195	784 H	473	152
Maine	278	42			54
Maryland	2,410 I	81	517		0
Massachusetts	1,209 J	158	361	669	0
Michigan	2,229				22
Minnesota	1,213	154	550	366	124
Mississippi	1,413	184			137
Missouri	1,377 K	142	767	259	114

Table 2 (cont.)

State	Total Pharmacies	Hospital/Institutional Pharmacies	Independent Community Pharmacies	Nonindependent Community Pharmacies (Four or More)	Out-of-State or Nonresident Pharmacies
Montana	290				0
Nebraska	588	95			84 L
Nevada	360	37	75	182	103
New Hampshire	252	45	65	134	0
New Jersey	2,054	162	1,263	626	
New Mexico	461	64	127 A	151 A	119
New York	4,461	498	2,275	1,577	0
North Carolina	2,011 F	157	629	930	82
North Dakota	332	49	181	20	82
Ohio	2,759 N	228	556	1,653	85
Oklahoma	1,022	91	931 A	A	102
Oregon	881	132	388	265	107
Pennsylvania	3,094	318			
Puerto Rico					
Rhode Island	207	24	70	113	26
South Carolina	1,228	197	422	540	79
South Dakota	269	38	173	58	0
Tennessee	1,637	216	814	560	47
Texas O	5,122 P	596	1,779	1,868	110
Utah	590	92	348 A	A	91
Vermont	137	18	137		0
Virginia	1,526				125
Washington	1,354	218 Q	480	532	124
West Virginia	572	87	183	302	93
Wisconsin	1,150				0
Wyoming	148	18	69	61	121
Totals	70,920	8,338	23,143	13,739	3,570

* Information provided directly from the state boards of pharmacy. Blanks indicate that information is not available.

Reprinted with permission from the 1996-97 National Association of Boards of Pharmacy *Survey of Pharmacy Law.*

Legend for Tables 1 and 2

A – Chains included in independent community pharmacies figure.
B – As of July 2, 1995.
C – As of July 1, 1995.
D – Approximately.
E – Plus 10 limited service and 45 parenteral admixture pharmacies.
F – In-state.
G – Includes 152 wholesalers, 5 manufacturers, and 4 provisional pharmacies.
H – Independent community pharmacies include 19 clinic, 12 correctional, 634 independent retail, 10 nuclear, 104 parenteral, and 5 other pharmacies.
I – Total includes other areas not listed: clinic, correctional, HMO, nursing home, IV, nuclear, research, and other.
J – Total also includes 12 home IV pharmacies, 11 LTCF pharmacies, and 1 mail-order pharmacy.
K – Includes 13 nursing home, 43 clinic, and 39 other pharmacies.
L – Nebraska "registers" out-of-state pharmacies.
M – Plus 335 who are practicing, but place is unknown.
N – Also licenses 237 nuclear, clinic, fluid therapy, mail-order, specialty, and pharmacies serving nursing homes only.
O – As of January 10, 1996.
P – Also licenses 769 nuclear, public health, clinic, ambulatory surgical center, and HMO pharmacies.
Q – Includes 114 hospital, 17 nursing home, 28 home infusion, 5 nuclear, 35 HMO, and 19 other pharmacies.

---

temporary pharmacists. As you will see, their careers are varied and ever changing. Chances are that the work these pharmacists are doing will surprise and intrigue you.

The next section of this chapter provides a thumbnail view of the profession. It talks about educational and licensing requirements, employment possibilities, advancement opportunities, salaries, and the employment outlook. Many of these topics are discussed in greater detail in later chapters of the *Companion*.

Pharmaceutical Care and Disease State Management

Pharmaceutical care. Disease state management. These are buzzwords of progressive pharmacy today. Learning about them will help you become more aware of how pharmacy has evolved to meet the challenges of today's health care environment.

Pharmaceutical care is the responsible provision of drug therapy for the purpose of achieving specific outcomes that improve a patient's quality of life.[1] The outcomes of pharmaceutical care are to cure disease, eliminate or reduce a patient's symptoms, arrest or slow a disease, or prevent disease.

What's important here is that the pharmacist focuses not on the medication but on optimizing use of that medication in a particular patient. Pharmaceutical care marks a dramatic departure from the traditional role of the pharmacist, which was restricted to "counting and pouring"—dispensing medications. Pharmaceutical care expands the responsibility of pharmacists. It places them in a new context that includes patients and other health professionals.

Pharmaceutical care, in other words, entails teamwork. Pharmacists work with nurses, physicians, pharmacy technicians, and other health professionals, as well as with patients, to develop a plan for managing the patient's disease. On this team, the pharmacist's unique expertise is the safe and effective use of medications.

Disease state management is the systematic review of a disease process (e.g., asthma, diabetes, or high blood pressure), the available treatment options, and the outcomes that those treatments may be expected to produce. It emphasizes the importance of patient education and compliance in the delivery of high-quality, cost-effective health care.

Disease state management programs may use protocols, guidelines, or algorithms that take the practitioner through a series of questions leading to a decision about the best care for a specific patient. Disease state management programs are developed in an interdisciplinary fashion and are research based. Well-designed disease state management programs not only improve patient outcomes but are also cost-effective.[2]

Pharmaceutical care and disease state management go hand in glove. Both are integral and evolving parts of contemporary pharmacy practice.

Pharmacist Profiles

Health care has changed a great deal in the past decade or so, and the pace of change continues. While cost-effectiveness efforts have in some cases revolutionized the way health care is delivered, it continues to be a growth field.

Moreover, pharmacists are keeping up with the times. Many are working in areas that did not exist 10 or 20 years ago. Consider the possibilities!

Pharmacist Entrepreneur

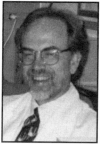

"Look for a market niche.... Get to know spreadsheets and computers backwards and forwards."

Dennis Cada

Dennis Cada, B.S., Pharm.D., Health Systems Editor, Facts & Comparisons, Dana Point, California

Cada worked for a year in community pharmacy after receiving his B.S. in pharmacy. He then went back to school for a Pharm.D. degree, after which he entered hospital pharmacy. He moved into the management track and became director of professional development for a hospital corporation. Searching for new areas to explore, he turned to computers and developed a system to computerize clinical functions "from the ground up." He became director of pharmacy at South Coast Hospital in 1982 and eventually was assigned administrative responsibility for several hospital units.

In 1986, Cada and a physician who was in charge of the hospital's pharmacy and therapeutics (P&T) committee joined forces to form a new company: Formulary Service, the Formulary Information Exchange (FIX). They spent two years developing their service, which is an electronic bulletin board that helps hospital pharmacists solve issues that arise from P&T committee deliberations. (The P&T committee decides which medications a hospital will stock. Those drugs are called the hospital formulary.) The project was a success. In 1990, Facts and Comparisons bought out the FIX, and Cada became its health-systems editor.

Cada is convinced that his single best career decision was to become involved with computers. "Get to know computers," he says, so that you can apply what these programs do to pharmacy practice. Students should have an "entrepreneurial spirit" and look for a market niche. They should continually be looking outside the profession to "systemwide" issues.

but his major focus has been pharmacy association management. For 20 years, Dee was the chief executive officer of a state pharmacy association. A brief hiatus from the field provided new "vision and detachment." He's now a consultant to pharmacy associations.

A pharmacist doesn't ordinarily set out to be a consultant, Dee notes. But if you've earned a good reputation in a well-defined field, sense that there's a niche for your services, and are somewhat of a risk taker, consultancy is a "natural." High levels of energy and self-discipline, the ability to work independently, organizational and communication skills, as well as a supportive family, are also prerequisites for success.

Dee believes that opportunities for newly licensed pharmacists are "unlimited." Hospital and community pharmacy continue to provide challenges; however, pharmacists don't have to limit themselves to traditional settings. Managed care, patient counseling, long-term care, systems analysis, and pharmacoeconomics will pose new challenges in the 21st century.

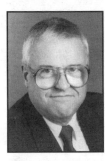

"Consultancy—there's no greater feeling of independence!"

Donald A. Dee

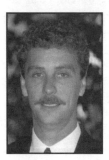

"Temper your instinct with experience, but don't forget: Your gut can lead your mind in some cases."

Michael J. Groh

Donald A. Dee, B.S., M.S., President, Donald A. Dee Consultants, Vienna, Virginia

Dee holds a bachelor's degree in pharmacy and a master's degree in pharmacy administration. He's worked in a community pharmacy,

Michael J. Groh, Pharm.D., President, Care Point, Inc., Charleston, South Carolina

Groh was an undergraduate student in the 1970s. He started out majoring in marine biology. Having become discouraged with that field, he sought advice from a friend who had just applied to pharmacy school. Groh consulted a pharmacist, who gave him some sound advice: "Get into clinical pharmacy!" Groh earned a Pharm.D. degree with emphasis in family practice from the Medical University of South Carolina. The program was unique in the country at that time.

Groh's initial experiences as a member of an outpatient health care team convinced him that pharmacists had much to share with physicians. He believed in pharmaceutical care before the term had been invented! Groh set up a business with several physician colleagues that enabled him to be reimbursed for counseling and drug information services. Later, Groh accepted a position at the Medical College of Virginia, where he was eventually promoted to associate director of ambulatory care. The next step in his career path was a position at National Data Corporation, where he was involved in the development and application of clinical databases.

Seeking yet another opportunity to apply his entrepreneurial, administrative, and technical skills, Groh, along with two pharmacist colleagues, founded Care Point, Inc. The organization provides computer software and training to pharmacists. Established only four years ago, Care Point now has a staff of 19, including 9 pharmacists.

Groh emphasizes the need to experiment with different positions before finding the one that's best. Today's students should concentrate from the start on disease state management and pharmaceutical care. For pharmacists with these skills, the future is a "golden age."

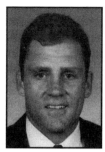

"Part of being a professional is being available to those you serve."

Brian J. Isetts

Brian J. Isetts, Ph.D., BCPS, President, Community Pharmacy Specialists, Red Wing, Minnesota

Isetts had a number of positions in his early career. He was in the clinical scientists program at the University of Minnesota and in community pharmacy. He also worked with the Minnesota Pharmacists Association. During this time, he became involved as a research associate with the Minnesota Pharmaceutical Care Project, which was centered at the University of Minnesota. "I saw pharmacy practice being revolutionized, and I wanted to be part of that revolution," Isetts recalls.

An opportunity soon presented itself. Isetts joined the staff of a large community pharmacy practice. In this clinical post, he helps patients identify and solve problems associated with medication use. The experience gained in this work, Isetts believes, helped him pass the examination to become a Board-Certified Pharmacotherapy Specialist (BCPS).

Isetts stresses that the practice of pharmacy doesn't always come easy. "Pharmaceutical care is difficult. You have to work hard. [Patient] noncompliance can be a big problem. You have to figure out a way to work with each patient." Flexibility is key; pharmaceutical care means being there for patients when they need you.

Pharmacy students have the responsibility for "moving the rest of the profession forward." That includes the difficult issue of reimbursement for cognitive services (that is, counseling and providing direct patient care). Each pharmacist has a role in improving practice. "If your goal is to help patients, find a good pharmacy and join it. Or find one that is 'almost there' and help take it to the next level." Isetts sees community pharmacists of the future participating in research to a greater extent. Areas to be explored include patient-outcome and quality-of-life studies.

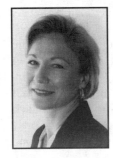

"Pharmacy is a profession you live for. It's not just an eight-hour-a-day job."

Anna Kowblansky

Anna Kowblansky, B.S., M.S., President, AK Consultants, Santa Barbara, California

Kowblansky has a bachelor of science degree in pharmacy and a master's degree in management of public services, with a specialty in health care. She's always been involved in pharmacy association work. As a student member of APhA, she participated in career days and other activities, believing that such involvement had a major role in "tying the real world" to pharmacy school.

Immediately after earning her B.S. degree, Kowblansky worked for a hospital pharmacy. She decided to enter association work and for a while worked for both the Illinois Council of Hospital Pharmacists and the Illinois Pharmacists Association. That led to a stint at APhA, where she worked with state relations and students. Then it was on to the Pharmaceutical Manufacturers Association, where she worked in state government affairs.

After moving to California a few years later, Kowblansky launched her career in consulting. Early clients included the California Pharmacists Association, the state board of pharmacy, and a pharmaceutical manufacturer.

Kowblansky advises students to "work hard and get as much experience as you can." Experience will help you find out what you like and don't like about a certain career. Networking is also essential; this is where organization membership really helps out.

She believes that the future belongs to pharmacists who can apply the knowledge they acquire in school and work as team players in the interest of patient care.

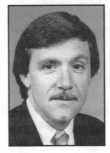

"Find a mentor. And learn all you can from this person."

Leo J. Sioris

Leo J. Sioris, Pharm.D., Director, Minnesota Regional Poison Control Center, and Assistant Professor of Pharmacy Practice, University of Minnesota College of Pharmacy, St. Paul, Minnesota

Before immigrating to the United States, Sioris's father was a pharmacist assistant in Greece. Son Leo enrolled in pharmacy school at the University of Minnesota. He came to his specialty—poison control—by a totally unplanned route. Having broken an ankle, he was unable to complete a scheduled rotation on the hospital wards and ended up being assigned to the Poison Control Center! After receiving his Pharm.D., Sioris worked in the center for several years and helped build many new programs. He was also on the staff of the Emergency Department.

Hospital downsizing forced Sioris to seek work elsewhere. He became a clinical pharmacist in a small hospital and remained a consultant to the poison center. Three years later, a new Poison Control Center was about to open in St. Paul. Sioris took the job, and he has remained there for the past 13 years.

The work is continually challenging. Among his chief duties is consulting with representatives of chemical manufacturers. This responsibility came about because Sioris recognized an opportunity to apply his pharmacy training to help these manufacturers decrease their liability, produce safer products, reduce patient risk, and comply with federal and state laws and regulations. Sioris has developed student externships and internships as well as a residency and fellowship in poison control.

Sioris emphasizes the importance of mentoring. Try to find a mentor who "excites you," he advises. Sioris himself had no mentor; as a result, he learned many lessons from the "school of hard knocks."

Sioris believes that the background students receive in pharmacy school prepares them for a wide range of careers. No other degree offers so much knowledge in "basic science, clinical science, business, and regulatory affairs." The key to success is to train not only in your area of specialty but also to cross-train. "The profession of pharmacy will move in any direction that enthusiastic and passionate pharmacists want it to."

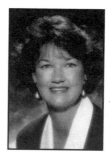

"To be successful, you have to be flexible. You also have to make some sacrifices—to pay your dues."

Donna Walker-Pulido

Donna Walker-Pulido, B.S., M.B.A., President, Pulido Walker Foundation, San Francisco, California

After graduating from pharmacy school, Walker-Pulido moved to Washington, D.C., to work at APhA headquarters. She was a staff member of the Association's student affairs office. Later, while working on a master's in business administration degree, she accepted a position at 3M Pharmaceuticals as a sales representative. The company was introducing a new product, and Walker-Pulido's business skills, combined with her knowledge of pharmacy, were invaluable.

She worked her way up quickly and became the first female district manager for 3M Pharmaceuticals. Realizing a long-held goal, she next became international marketing manager for the company. In the years that followed, she was promoted to marketing operations manager and, finally, to director of sales and marketing for 3M's telecommunications firm.

When her husband was offered a promising position in San Francisco, Walker-Pulido decided to make a major life change as well. She is now president of the Pulido Walker Foundation, which focuses on developing entrepreneurialism in children.

Walker-Pulido recommends "following your dream" and "listening to those around you." It was listening to her mentor that led her to enter an M.B.A. program. Flexibility and the willingness to compromise are also essential. For example, a lateral career move is okay, she says, if it helps move you toward your goal.

Pharmacists who practice in the 21st century must be able to apply technology to their profession. Through telecommunications and telemedicine, for example, pharmacists may even be able to make house calls. Improved communications will offer pharmacists new opportunities for monitoring patient care and improving patient compliance.

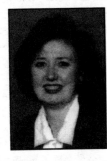

"Get enough work experience to find out what you like and dislike, what you want to do and what you don't want to do."

Lynn F. Williams

Lynn F. Williams, B.S., President, Solutions, Tampa, Florida

Williams started out majoring in math and science. She then switched to pharmacy and worked as a pharmacy technician as an undergraduate. Because she enjoyed working with older patients, she took a position with a company as staff pharmacist in a nursing home.

The business grew, and she grew with it. After the company was bought out, she was named a regional manager and then vice president for operations for the southeastern United States. During that time, she also gained experience as a surveyor in home infusion and long-term care for the Joint Commission on Accreditation of Healthcare Organizations.

Williams left the company in 1991 to start Solutions, a business that consults with companies providing home infusion therapy. The company soon branched out to offer training for pharmacists and pharmaceutical representatives. Williams has developed training programs in areas such as reimbursement, legislative trends in long-term care, and disease state management.

While her responsibilities as president of Solutions keep her busy, Williams makes time for other activities. To maintain patient contact, she does consulting in a long-term facility. Her longstanding contributions to association work were capped by a recent term as chairman of the board of the American Society of Consultant Pharmacists.

Williams's career path, as she puts it, led her from focusing directly on the patient to focusing on management, in which she "impacts patients by impacting others." She emphasizes the importance of mentoring in career development. Association membership is also important because of the contacts and networking opportunities it affords.

Clinical care is key to the future of pharmacy, Williams believes. Pharmacist involvement must be continuous, not episodic. Technology can make prospective care and disease state management possible. Finally, pharmacists must increasingly document the economic impact of the services they provide.

Practicing Pharmacist

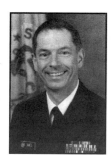

"Public Health Service pharmacy ... allows mobility, variety, and access to progressive clinical practice."

Timothy W. Ames

Timothy W. Ames, B.A., B.S., M.P.H., Regulatory Health Project Manager, Office of Generic Drugs, Food and Drug Administration (FDA), Rockville, Maryland

Ames earned a bachelor's in chemistry before entering pharmacy school at Wayne State University. His preceptor at Wayne State got him interested in the progressive pharmacy services offered by the Indian Health Service (IHS). He applied for a commission in the Public Health Service (PHS), in the hope of eventually being assigned to the IHS. He accepted a commission in the PHS; with it came the opportunity to do a residency at a hospital in New York City. He stayed in New York for two years. From there, he was assigned to duty in Hawaii.

Ames made it to the IHS several years later. He was a clinical pharmacist for a 125-bed hospital that cared for Navajo and Hopi Native Americans.

In 1984, Ames traveled back east to join the National Institutes of Health (NIH) as a staff pharmacist. He then moved to the NIH pharmaceutical development center. Along the way, he earned a master's degree in public health from the Johns Hopkins University.

Ames joined the FDA in 1992 as a consumer safety officer in the Center for Drug Evaluation and Research. He facilitates the review of abbreviated new drug applications. He is also the chief pharmacist for the PHS Disaster Medical Assistance Team. In this capacity, he deploys pharmacists in areas that have been declared disaster areas by the Federal Emergency Management Agency.

Ames believes that the federal government offers many exciting opportunities for pharmacists in clinical work as well as management. In many cases, he notes, exposure to the PHS may begin with participation in COSTEP, a 10-week summer training experience offered to junior and senior pharmacy students. He urges young pharmacists to consider a PHS career.

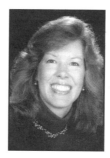

"Fellowships can put you on the 'fast track' with physicians and in academia."

Grace Hayes

Grace Hayes, Pharm.D., Clinical Pharmacist, Atascadero State Hospital, Atascadero, California

Hayes worked in a chain drugstore while she was a student. She also worked in an independent pharmacy. Another early experience as an intern at Atascadero State Hospital, however, convinced her that psychiatric pharmacy was the career for her.

What should a student who is interested in this specialty do? Develop good communications skills, for one thing. They are especially helpful for pharmacists who specialize in psychopharmacy. She also stresses the need for on-the-job training, patient contact, and a good mentor. An ambulatory residency can provide a broad base of skills. The best way to "jump start" your career? A residency or fellowship in psychiatric pharmacy. Fellowship experience, Hayes believes, is a definite asset if you plan to work on a team with physicians.

Hayes sees several trends on the horizon. First, pharmacists will become integrated with the health care team. Admittedly, it's a slow process. Some pharmacists may find it best to have broad-based skills; others will carve out a distinctive niche in areas such as homeopathy. Hayes foresees the demise of chain drugstores that do not offer pharmaceutical care. Community pharmacists who provide health information centers, by contrast, will thrive.

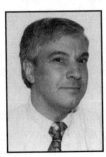

"Find the practice you want, and the rewards will come."

John Parisi

John Parisi, B.S., Owner, Ivery & Dudley Pharmacy, Winsted, Connecticut

Parisi received his bachelor's degree in 1971. Shortly thereafter, he and two colleagues purchased a community pharmacy. He slowly bought out his two business partners over the next few years.

Parisi's practice was "fairly typical" until a few years ago, when he became energized by a presentation on how pharmacists can manage the care of patients with asthma. He transformed his pharmacy into a health education center. This required not only remodeling his store but developing a totally new mindset. He's had remarkable success.

Parisi put together a program entitled "Together, We Can Manage Your Asthma." He's now trained 150 people in Winsted, a town of 11,000. He offers free blood pressure screening and glucose measurement every Monday. He's become a certified diabetes educator and has developed a home management class on diabetes.

As an additional service to his patients with diabetes, he's established referral links with an area dietitian, optometrist, and podiatrist.

Today's pharmacists must "embrace change" and know what they want to do. "Don't sell out for a few thousand dollars," he advises. In other words, don't take a position only because it offers a higher salary than another.

Parisi sees many opportunities for young pharmacists in health centers such as his. To continue the "ownership process," he encourages students to get to know independent pharmacy owners.

The keys to success in independent pharmacy? "Entrepreneurial spirit, the ability to communicate, and a liking for people."

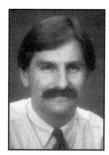

"The decision to do a residency in critical-care pharmacy was the best career move I ever made."

Greg Susla

Greg Susla, B.S., Pharm.D., Critical Care Pharmacist, National Institutes of Health, Bethesda, Maryland

Susla's dad was a pharmacist, and Greg worked in a community pharmacy during his adolescence and pharmacy school. He earned his undergraduate pharmacy degree in 1980. After graduation, he returned to his hometown to enter community practice.

That experience lasted only three months. Next, Susla took a position in a local hospital. He realized he'd found his niche. After working for a few years, he returned to school to earn a Pharm.D. degree. He also completed a residency in critical care pharmacy. He moved on to a post in a larger hospital and then joined the pharmacy staff at the National Institutes of Health (NIH) in the mid-1980s.

Susla says that the specialty residency was especially worthwhile because it enabled him to obtain a position at NIH. Each job, however, made an invaluable contribution to his knowledge base. For example, his early work as a pharmacy technician helped reinforce the classroom knowledge to which he was exposed in pharmacy school; it made that knowledge "real world."

Pharmacy students, Susla believes, should be "well rounded." Grades are important, but on-the-job experience and involvement in association work also produce payoffs. Postgraduate work fills in the gaps in pharmacy education and gives you special skills.

Susla is optimistic about the future. Greater involvement in patient welfare, including service as a patient advocate, is the wave of the future for pharmacy.

Association Management

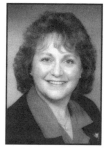

"Don't be afraid to fail, especially if you can learn from it. Create the future you want."

Phyllis Moret

Phyllis Moret, B.S., Associate Executive Director, American Society of Consultant Pharmacists (ASCP), Alexandria, Virginia

Moret began her career at age 13—as a "soda jerk" in a local pharmacy. After graduating from pharmacy school, she became a hospital pharmacist. She then returned to her hometown in Mississippi where she worked in a community pharmacy and in another hospital pharmacy.

Her next career move was to the Mississippi Pharmacists Association. She served as executive director of this organization for 13 years. She then turned to association work at the national level, working briefly at APhA before joining ASCP.

Moret claims to have learned a lot from each of her positions.

From the community pharmacist in her hometown, she learned about interpersonal relations and how the judicious use of humor can "ease a bad situation or interaction." She learned about administration from a director of hospital pharmacy. Both of these individuals, she gratefully recalls, were her mentors.

She advises students to "think outside the typical pharmacy career box." They should focus on basic skills such as writing and speaking, which are helpful in any setting. Computer literacy is essential.

The future of pharmacy is for pharmacists who "forget how to put pills in a bottle." Pharmacists' value is in "having information and knowing how to manipulate that information. It is also caring for people."

Managed Care Pharmacy

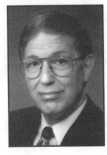

"Don't be afraid to be a trailblazer."

David Angaran

David Angaran, B.S., M.S., Vice President for Clinical Training and Education, Medco Containment Services, Columbus, Ohio

Angaran earned a bachelor of science degree in pharmacy and a master's degree in hospital pharmacy. He spent six years on the faculty of the University of Wisconsin School of Pharmacy and then moved to the University of Minnesota, where he taught and practiced critical care pharmacy. He joined Medco in 1995.

A good position, Angaran believes, is one in which you acquire knowledge and skills that you can apply to your next position. His present position centers on advancing the practice of pharmaceutical care. He evaluates activities involved with delivery of pharmaceutical care, designs tools to measure and improve the outcome of pharmaceutical services, and develops training modules to support pharmaceutical care.

What does today's pharmacist need? A sense of adventure and belief in oneself, Angaran says. "The places where you can make the most difference are the places where nobody has been before." This means that you must not only go beyond the minimum requirements set forth on your job description but also be accountable for your actions.

What will tomorrow's pharmacists need? Angaran feels there is a great future for pharmacists in information systems. Success in this area requires more than technical know-how. If the people involved with technology don't communicate with one another, the potential of information systems cannot be realized.

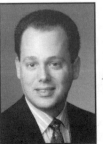

"Drill down to find the jewel in different practice settings."

Michael Manolakis

Michael Manolakis, Pharm.D., Senior Director of Product Development, Value Rx, Minneapolis, Minnesota

Manolakis did his undergraduate work in pharmacy at the University of Southern California. His first position was in a chain drug store. His interactions with patients in that setting, combined with an emerging concern about issues related to the treatment of acquired immunodeficiency syndrome (AIDS), led him to pursue a doctor of philosophy degree in biomedical ethics. While working toward his Ph.D., Manolakis accepted a position with a pharmacy benefits management company. The field was new at the time, and Manolakis was able to gain experience in a promising area. His title was administrator and developer of case management. The work was stimulating. It involved conferences with other health professionals and "robust discussions" of the treatment of disease. Part of his work entailed evaluating certificates of medical necessity, a responsibility for which his background in ethics was invaluable.

Manolakis advises young pharmacists to get as much training and work experience as possible. "Take a chance, follow your dream. You can't always expect a payoff, but the results can often be rewarding." Manolakis also counsels students to take advantage of networking and mentoring opportunities. Students should certainly look for opportunities within the profession; at the same time, "look beyond pharmacy to the larger field of health care."

Pharmacists of the future should consider their pharmacy degree as a building block that will facilitate involvement with an increasingly integrated health care system. The spectrum of opportunity is "any place in which drug therapy management is 'part of the picture.'"

Pharmacy ABC's

Educational Requirements

Pharmacy offers two entry-level degrees: the bachelor of science (B.S.) and the doctor of pharmacy (Pharm.D.). Students can earn a B.S. in five years; the Pharm.D. requires an additional year of study. Pharmacy degrees are offered in the nation's 79 schools and colleges of pharmacy.

Some pharmacists go on to earn master's or doctor of philosophy degrees in related fields. Some earn dual degrees (e.g., in pharmacy and law or in pharmacy and business administration).

Many pharmacists also participate in pharmacy residency and fellowship programs. Residency programs are offered both in general and specialty practice. Fellowships are geared primarily to individuals whose goal is a career in research.

For more information on degrees and pharmacy schools, see Chapters 2 and 3. Information on residencies and fellowships appears in Chapter 6.

Licensure

Before entering practice, pharmacy graduates must pass a national licensure examination and meet additional requirements in the states in which they intend to practice.

Yearly relicensure is required. Requirements are state specific.

To be relicensed, a pharmacist must satisfactorily complete a specified number of continuing-education units.

For more information about licensure, see Chapter 7.

Certification

Pharmacists who specialize in a field (e.g., psychopharmacy, nutrition support, or cancer treatment) may voluntarily seek board certification by sitting for a specialty examination. Board certification is overseen by the Board of Pharmaceutical Specialties. For more information, contact the Board of Pharmaceutical Specialties, 2215 Constitution Avenue, N.W., Washington, DC 20037-2985. Telephone (202) 429-7591.

Earnings

Pharmacist salaries depend on experience, training, geographic location, and work setting. Because there are so many variables, salary ranges are broad. For example, annual salaries of entry-level pharmacists in community pharmacies, hospital pharmacies, and pharmaceutical manufacturing firms range from $40,000 to $70,000. Managers' salaries range from $50,000 to $70,000.

New pharmacy graduates with a B.S. degree who are hired by the federal government earn between $28,000 to $36,000 (grade GS-9) and $34,000 to $44,000 (grade GS-11).

At pharmacy schools, annual salaries are approximately $80,000 for full professors, $62,000 for associate professors, and $53,000 for assistant professors.

Long-term care consultant pharmacists may earn upwards of $75,000.

Salaried pharmacists receive fringe benefits, including sick leave, vacation leave, medical and life insurance, and a pension or profit-sharing plan, among others. Self-employed pharmacists may have greater freedom than their salaried colleagues, but they also have substantially more responsibilities. Self-employed pharmacists must, for example, purchase or lease properties, stock medications and supplies, hire personnel, and pay overhead expenses.

Advancement Opportunities

Pharmacists working in community pharmacies may eventually become managers. Owners of independent pharmacies with the necessary financial resources can eventually own several stores.

Pharmacists working for the federal government receive regularly scheduled advances in grade level with corresponding salary increases. Pharmacists employed by research and manufacturing companies may rise to high-level administrative or research positions. Hospital pharmacists may advance by becoming specialists or by being promoted to management positions. In these positions, they may oversee several hospital divisions, including the pharmacy.

Pharmacists in colleges may advance from instructor to professor and, perhaps, to dean.

Will There Be a Job for Me in the Year 2002? In 2022?

The employment outlook for pharmacists is good. Why? The U.S. population is growing—and aging. More and more medications are being developed, and drug therapy is becoming more complex. Many prescription drugs are being moved to nonprescription status. This trend offers pharmacists new opportunities in patient education. What's more, the public is becoming increasingly health conscious. As managed care poses restrictions on use of the health care system, many patients will increasingly rely on their pharmacist as an accessible and informed health professional.

If you've read the pharmacist interviews that begin this chapter, you'll realize, however, that maintaining viability in today's economy will require flexibility, imagination, and a bit of daring.

A B.S. or Pharm.D. degree is just the beginning. You'll have many more learning opportunities ahead. Each position, as the pharmacist profiles show, is in itself a learning experience. You'll also have to complete a minimum number of continuing-education units annually to qualify for relicensure. But more important, you'll have to keep pace with the changes that will continue to occur all around you in computer technology, in health and pharmaceutical research, in management—and elsewhere.

Keep your options open, keep learning and growing, and the possibilities are indeed limitless.

References

1. Hepler CD, Strand LM. Opportunities and responsibilities in pharmaceutical care. Am J Hosp Pharm. 1990;47:533-43.
2. Armstrong EP, Langley PC. Disease management programs. Am J Health-Syst Pharm. 1996;53:53-8.

Chapter 2: Is Pharmacy the Career for You

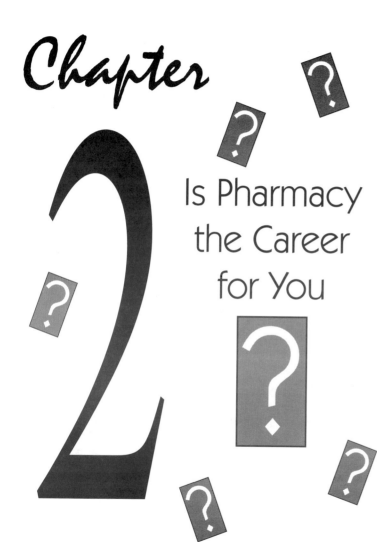

Introduction

You've always done well in science and math. You're interested in helping people. Health careers have always been appealing. As a child, you dreamed about becoming a physician. As a former hospital patient, you remember the compassion of a nurse.

Maybe you've already thought about a career in pharmacy, maybe you have not. But if the descriptions above sound a lot like you, then you share the characteristics of many of today's pharmacy students.

Here are some real-life examples. Each is now a pharmacy student.

• Marci entered pharmacy school because she "likes science and people." Her brother is a pharmacist.

• Charlotte lives in a small town. When her uncle was dying of cancer, she became close to the pharmacist who managed his home care. She was impressed by the pharmacist's knowledge as well as his caring attitude. During that time, the pharmacist "became like a member of the family." He was always available to answer their questions.

• Darrell had always dreamed of a career as a health professional. He assumed he'd become a physician. Pharmacist friends convinced him that they had a great deal more patient contact than doctors do. Once he'd looked into it, Darrell agreed.

• Jim B. wanted "flexibility." He also wanted a career in which he could interact with professionals of other disciplines.

• Jim M. was attracted by the starting salaries offered by the pharmacy profession. He liked math and science but did not want to do basic research.

• Melissa also liked science and math. In addition, she was a sports enthusiast. She decided to go into pharmacy and to focus on sports medicine. Her goal? "A spot on the Olympic Committee."

• Timothy had his sights set on a career of government service—either in the military or the Public Health Service. The more he heard about pharmaceutical care, the better it sounded.

How to Start

If you think you might be interested in a career in pharmacy, talk with your school or campus guidance counselor.

Equally important, talk with a pharmacist! Part-time or summer employment in a pharmacy may help you decide. Community pharmacies offer positions for sales clerks, stock clerks, word processors, and cashiers. Hospital pharmacies hire laboratory helpers and pharmacy couriers.

While you're on the job, be as observant as possible. What's the atmosphere like? Can you see yourself enjoying and being challenged by a pharmacist's duties? Have lunch or take a break with the pharmacists. Ask them about their education and training and about their satisfaction with their work.

Pathways to Pharmacy

As you continue to explore what pharmacy has to offer, you'll want to obtain as much information as you can about pharmacy education. You'll find that the education of a pharmacist is a bit more complicated than that of some other professionals.

In fact, students enter pharmacy school by a number of routes. Three are most common.

• Most students enter pharmacy school after completing one or two years of undergraduate work at a four-year college or junior college. This is called preprofessional or prepharmacy study.

• Some students enter pharmacy school immediately after leaving high school. Such students can earn a Pharm.D. degree within six years of high school graduation. Many pharmacy schools, however, do not accept students directly from high school.

• Some students enter pharmacy school after earning a bachelor's degree. Such students are generally awarded degrees in biology, chemistry, biochemistry, or a related field.

None of these approaches has particular advantages or disadvantages. The main effect is that you, the student, have a choice. As soon as you've begun to think about entering pharmacy school, it's a good idea to check with the schools in which you are interested. In this way, you'll be able to familiarize yourself with their particular admissions policies.

Which Degree Is Right for Me?

The study of pharmacy generally leads to one of two entry-level degrees: a bachelor of science (B.S.) in pharmacy or a doctor of pharmacy (Pharm.D.) degree. You may also earn a postgraduate master's degree (M.S.) or doctor of philosophy degree (Ph.D.) in a pharmacy-related field. (The letters R.Ph., which appear after a pharmacist's name, refer to licensure and have nothing to do with degree status. They are an abbreviation for registered pharmacist.)

B.S. and Pharm.D. Degrees

For many years, the B.S. was the standard entry-level pharmacy degree in this country. The B.S. requires five years of study. In the mid-1970s, schools of pharmacy began offering a second degree, the Pharm.D. (The trend toward the Pharm.D. degree began even earlier in California, where it has been offered since the late 1950s.) Pharm.D. candidates are required to complete all courses required of B.S. pharmacists. In addition, they take courses in diseases and drug therapy management. They also must complete additional courses in areas such as pharmacokinetics (the science of how medications behave in a living organism). The Pharm.D. is a six-year course of study. The number of pharmacists who hold Pharm.D. degrees is growing. In 1994–1995, 30% of all entry-level degrees were Pharm.D.s.

Today, most schools of pharmacy offer both degrees. By the year 2000, however, schools may offer only the Pharm.D. This is because in 1992 the American Association of Colleges of Pharmacy (AACP) voted to establish the Pharm.D. as the sole entry-level degree for the profession. AACP believes that pharmacy training beyond the B.S. degree is essential because of the increasing complexity of health care and drug therapy management.

M.S. and Ph.D. Degrees

B.S.- or Pharm.D.-level pharmacists who wish to pursue a particular field of study in depth may enter master's or Ph.D. programs. Master's programs are available in hospital administration, business administration, clinical pharmacy, public health, and other areas. Training at the Ph.D. level is available in all the pharmaceutical sciences as well as in social and administrative pharmacy. Students who pursue a Ph.D. are interested in research and in the application of science to practice.

For more information about graduate programs in pharmacy, see Chapter 3.

Admission Requirements

Personal Qualifications

The best pharmacists are both scientists and humanists. They have excellent analytic, critical-thinking, and problem-solving skills. High academic ability is needed; above average grades in math and science are recommended. At the same time, pharmacists need strong interpersonal skills. They must enjoy working with and helping people. High ethical standards are required.

Pharmacy appeals to both women and men. During the past decade, half of all pharmacy degrees have been awarded to women.

A final qualification is a love of learning. Pharmacists must be lifelong learners. The rapid pace of change in health care demands it.

Educational Qualifications

If you plan to transfer to pharmacy school after two years of prepharmacy work, you should enroll in courses in chemistry, biology, physics, calculus, anatomy and physiology, social science, economics, and English during your prepharmacy years.

Some colleges of pharmacy require that applicants take the Pharmacy College Admission Test (PCAT). Check with the admissions office of the schools in which you are interested to see if this is a requirement.

Choosing a Pharmacy School

There are 79 accredited schools and colleges of pharmacy in the nation (see Appendix A at end of chapter). The schools differ substantially in many respects; for this reason, you will want to do solid research to determine the one that's best for you.

Factors to Consider in Selecting a Pharmacy School

What questions should you ask in evaluating a school or college of pharmacy? Think about the following:

Location. Do you want an urban environment or do you prefer a more rural setting? The West Coast or the East Coast? Or somewhere in between?

Enrollment. Are you more comfortable in a small school or a large one? For a benchmark, consider that enrollment in U.S. schools of pharmacy in the fall of 1995 ranged from 125 to 1,417.

Admissions Policies. Forty-four schools require that applicants take the PCAT examination. Other admission policies relate to high school and undergraduate grade point averages, extracurricular activities, and work experience.

Degrees Offered. Virtually all schools offer both the B.S. and Pharm.D. degrees. Many schools of pharmacy also offer dual degrees that allow you to study concurrently for a B.S or Pharm.D. and another degree. If you already know that you're interested in combining two fields, this can save you time (and money).

The most common dual degree is a Pharm.D. plus a master's of business administration (M.B.A.), which is offered by 10 schools. Other options include a Pharm.D. and law degree (J.D.). Check with the admissions office about dual-degree possibilities.

Acceptance Rate. At the interview, you may want to inquire about the ratio of applications received to the number of students accepted. This currently ranges from about 1.27:1 to 8.24:1.

Accreditation Status. Schools of pharmacy are accredited by the American Council on Pharmaceutical Education (ACPE). To determine a school's continued eligibility for accreditation, ACPE reviews each school's curriculum every few years. It also reviews the size of the faculty, faculty credentials, and the physical facility.

Tuition Rates

Tuition rates vary. For public, state-supported schools, the single greatest difference is between rates offered to students who reside in the state and out-of-state rates. In 1997-98, first-year tuition and fees for a B.S. program ranged from $1,480 to $19,065 (in state) and from $3,565 to $19,065 (out-of-state).

For the Pharm.D. degree, the costs ranged from $1,512 to $26,805 (in state) to $3,570 to $26,805 (out of state).

Additional Resources

For more guidance on selecting a school, consult *Pharmacy School Admission Requirements*, available from AACP for $25 plus a $3 handling charge. Telephone (703) 739-2330.

Appendix A

U.S. Schools and Colleges of Pharmacy

ALABAMA

School of Pharmacy
Auburn University
Auburn, AL 36849-5501
Phone: (334) 844-8351

McWhorter School of Pharmacy
Samford University
800 Lakeshore Drive
Birmingham, AL 35229
Phone: (205) 870-2820

ARIZONA

College of Pharmacy
The University of Arizona
P.O. Box 210207
Tucson, AZ 85721-0207
Phone: (520) 626-1427

ARKANSAS

College of Pharmacy
University of Arkansas for Medical Sciences
4301 West Markham - Slot 522
Little Rock, AR 72205-7122
Phone: (501) 686-5557

CALIFORNIA

School of Pharmacy
University of California
S-926
San Francisco, CA 94143-0446
Phone: (415) 476-1925

School of Pharmacy
University of the Pacific
3601 Pacific Avenue
Stockton, CA 95211
Phone: (209) 946-2561

School of Pharmacy
University of Southern California
1985 Zonal Avenue
Los Angeles, CA 90033-1086
Phone: (213) 342-1369

College of Pharmacy
Western University of Health Sciences
College Plaza
309 East Second Street
Pomona, CA 91766-1889
Phone: (909) 469-5500

COLORADO

School of Pharmacy
University of Colorado Health Sciences Center
C238
4200 East Ninth Avenue
Denver, CO 80262-0238
Phone: (303) 270-5055

CONNECTICUT

School of Pharmacy
The University of Connecticut
Box U92/372 Fairfield Road
Storrs, CT 06269-2092
Phone: (860) 486-2129

DISTRICT of COLUMBIA

College of Pharmacy and
Pharmacal Sciences
Howard University
2300 4th Street, NW
Washington, DC 20059
Phone: (202) 806-6530

FLORIDA

College of Pharmacy and Pharmacal Sciences
Florida Agricultural and Mechanical University
Tallahassee, FL 32307-3800
Phone: (904) 599-3593

College of Pharmacy
Nova Southeastern University
3200 South University Drive
Ft. Lauderdale, FL 33328
Phone: (954) 723-1300

College of Pharmacy
University of Florida
Box 100484
Health Science Center
Gainesville, FL 32610-0484
Phone: (352) 392-9713

GEORGIA

Southern School of Pharmacy
Mercer University
3001 Mercer University Drive
Atlanta, GA 30341-4155
Phone: (770) 986-3300

College of Pharmacy
University of Georgia
Athens, GA 30602-2351
Phone: (706) 542-1911

IDAHO

College of Pharmacy
Campus Box 8288
Idaho State University
Pocatello, ID 83209-8288
Phone: (208) 236-2175

ILLINOIS

Chicago College of Pharmacy
Midwestern University
555 31st Street
Downers Grove, IL 60515-1235
Phone: (630) 971-6417

College of Pharmacy (M/C 874)
University of Illinois at Chicago
833 South Wood Street
Chicago, IL 60612-7230
Phone: (312) 996-7240

INDIANA

College of Pharmacy and Health Sciences
Butler University
4600 Sunset Avenue
Indianapolis, IN 46208
Phone: (317) 940-9322

School of Pharmacy and Pharmacal Sciences
1330 Heine Pharmacy Building
Purdue University
West Lafayette, IN 47907-1330
Phone: (317) 494-1357

IOWA

College of Pharmacy and Health Sciences
Drake University
2507 University Avenue
Des Moines, IA 50311-4505
Phone: (515) 271-2172

College of Pharmacy
The University of Iowa
Iowa City, IA 52242
Phone: (319) 335-8794

KANSAS

School of Pharmacy
University of Kansas
2056 Malott
Lawrence, KS 66045-2500
Phone: (913) 864-3591

KENTUCKY

College of Pharmacy
University of Kentucky
Rose Street - Pharmacy Building
Lexington, KY 40536-0082
Phone: (606) 257-2737

LOUISIANA

School of Pharmacy
Northeast Louisiana University
700 University Avenue
Monroe, LA 71209-0470
Phone: (318) 342-1600

25

Appendix A (cont.)

College of Pharmacy
Xavier University of Louisiana
7325 Palmetto Street
New Orleans, LA 70125
Phone: (504) 483-7424

MARYLAND

School of Pharmacy
University of Maryland
20 North Pine Street
Baltimore, MD 21201-1180
Phone: (410) 706-7650

MASSACHUSETTS

Massachusetts College of Pharmacy and
Allied Health Sciences
179 Longwood Avenue
Boston, MA 02115-5896
Phone: (617) 732-2800

Bouve College of Pharmacy and
Health Sciences
Northeastern University
360 Huntington Avenue
Boston, MA 02115
Phone: (617) 373-3321

MICHIGAN

College of Pharmacy
Ferris State University
220 Ferris Drive
Big Rapids, MI 49307-2740
Phone: (616) 592-2254

College of Pharmacy
The University of Michigan
Ann Arbor, MI 48109-1065
Phone: (313) 764-7312

College of Pharmacy and
Allied Health Professions
Wayne State University
105 Shapero Hall
Detroit, MI 48202-3489
Phone: (313) 577-1574

MINNESOTA

College of Pharmacy
University of Minnesota
5-130 Weaver-Densford Hall
308 Harvard Street SE
Minneapolis, MN 55455-0343
Phone: (612) 624-1900

MISSISSIPPI

School of Pharmacy
The University of Mississippi
University, MS 38677-9814
Phone: (601) 232-7265

MISSOURI

St. Louis College of Pharmacy
4588 Parkview Place
St. Louis, MO 63110-1088
Phone: (314) 367-8700

School of Pharmacy
University of Missouri - Kansas City
5005 Rockhill Road
Kansas City, MO 64110-2499
Phone: (816) 235-1609

MONTANA

School of Pharmacy and
Allied Health Sciences
University of Montana
Missoula, MT 59812-1075
Phone: (406) 243-4621

NEBRASKA

School of Pharmacy and
Allied Health Professions
Creighton University
2500 California Plaza
Omaha, NE 68178
Phone: (402) 280-2950

College of Pharmacy
University of Nebraska
600 South 42nd Street
Omaha, NE 68198-6000
Phone: (402) 559-4333

NEW JERSEY

College of Pharmacy
Rutgers University
The State University of New Jersey
P.O. Box 789
Piscataway, NJ 08855-0789
Phone: (908) 445-2666

NEW MEXICO

College of Pharmacy
Health Sciences Center
The University of New Mexico
Albuquerque, NM 87131-1066
Phone: (505) 277-2461

NEW YORK

Albany College of Pharmacy
Union University
106 New Scotland
Albany, NY 12208
Phone: (518) 445-7200

Arnold and Marie Schwartz
College of Pharmacy and Health Sciences
Long Island University
75 DeKalb Avenue at University Plaza
Brooklyn, NY 11201
Phone: (718) 488-1060

College of Pharmacy and
Allied Health Professions
St. John's University
Grand Central and Utopia Parkways
Jamaica, NY 11439
Phone: (718) 990-6275

School of Pharmacy
SUNY at Buffalo
C126 Cooke-Hochstetter Complex
Buffalo, NY 14260-1200
Phone: (716) 645-2823

NORTH CAROLINA

School of Pharmacy
Campbell University
P.O. Box 1090
Buies Creek, NC 27506
Phone: (910) 893-1685

School of Pharmacy
University of North Carolina
Beard Hall CB#7360
Chapel Hill, NC 27599-7360
Phone: (919) 966-1121

NORTH DAKOTA

College of Pharmacy
Box 5505
North Dakota State University
Fargo, ND 58105
Phone: (701) 231-7456

OHIO

College of Pharmacy
Ohio Northern University
Ada, OH 45810
Phone: (419) 772-2275

College of Pharmacy
The Ohio State University
500 West 12th Avenue
Columbus, OH 43210-1291
Phone: (614) 292-2266

College of Pharmacy
University of Cincinnati Medical Center
P.O. Box 670004
Cincinnati, OH 45267-0004
Phone: (513) 558-3784

College of Pharmacy
University of Toledo
2801 West Bancroft Street
Toledo, OH 43606-3390
Phone: (419) 530-2019

OKLAHOMA

School of Pharmacy
Southwestern Oklahoma State University
100 Campus Drive
Weatherford, OK 73096
Phone: (405) 774-3105

College of Pharmacy
University of Oklahoma
P.O. Box 26901
Oklahoma City, OK 73190-5040
Phone: (405) 271-6484

OREGON

College of Pharmacy
Oregon State University
Pharmacy Building 203
Corvallis, OR 97331-3507
Phone: (541) 737-3424

Appendix A (cont.)

PENNSYLVANIA

Mylan School of Pharmacy
Duquesne University
Pittsburgh, PA 15282
Phone: (412) 396-6380

School of Pharmacy
Philadelphia College of Pharmacy and Science
600 South 43rd Street
Philadelphia, PA 19140-4495
Phone: (215) 596-8870

School of Pharmacy
Temple University of the Commonwealth System of Higher Education
3307 North Broad Street
Philadelphia, PA 19140
Phone: (215) 707-4990

School of Pharmacy
University of Pittsburgh
1106 Salk Hall
Pittsburgh, PA 15261
Phone: (412) 648-8579

School of Pharmacy
Wilkes University
Wilkes-Barre, PA 18766
Phone: (717) 831-4280

PUERTO RICO

School of Pharmacy
University of Puerto Rico
P.O. Box 365067
San Juan, PR 00936-5067
Phone: (787) 758-2525, ext. 5400

RHODE ISLAND

College of Pharmacy
University of Rhode Island
Kingston, RI 02881-0809
Phone: (401) 874-2761

SOUTH CAROLINA

College of Pharmacy
Medical University of South Carolina
171 Ashley Avenue
Charleston, SC 29425-2301
Phone: (803) 792-3115

College of Pharmacy
University of South Carolina
Columbia, SC 29208
Phone: (803) 777-4151

SOUTH DAKOTA

College of Pharmacy
South Dakota State University
Box 2202C
Brookings, SD 57007-0099
Phone: (605) 688-6197

TENNESSEE

College of Pharmacy
University of Tennessee
847 Monroe Avenue
Suite 200
Memphis, TN 38163
Phone: (901) 448-6036

TEXAS

College of Pharmacy and Health Sciences
Texas Southern University
3100 Cleburne
Houston, TX 77004
Phone: (713) 313-7164

School of Pharmacy
Texas Tech University
1300 South Coulter Street
Amarillo, TX 79106
Phone: (806) 354-5463

College of Pharmacy
University of Houston
4800 Calhoun
Houston, TX 77204-5511
Phone: (713) 743-1300

College of Pharmacy
University of Texas at Austin
Austin, TX 78712-1074
Phone: (512) 471-1737

UTAH

College of Pharmacy
University of Utah
Salt Lake City, UT 84112
Phone: (801) 581-6731

VIRGINIA

School of Pharmacy
Shenandoah University
1460 University Drive
Winchester, VA 22601
Phone: (540) 665-1282

School of Pharmacy
Virginia Commonwealth University
MCV Campus - Box 980581
410 North 12th Street
Richmond, VA 23298-0581
Phone: (804) 828-3000

WASHINGTON

School of Pharmacy
University of Washington
H-364 Health Sciences Center
Box 357631
Seattle, WA 98195
Phone: (206) 543-2453

College of Pharmacy
Washington State University
P.O. Box 646510
Pullman, WA 99164-6510
Phone: (509) 335-8664

WEST VIRGINIA

School of Pharmacy
West Virginia University
HSC 1136 HSN
P.O. Box 9500
Morgantown, WV 26506-9500
Phone: (304) 293-5101

WISCONSIN

School of Pharmacy
University of Wisconsin - Madison
425 North Charter Street
Madison, WI 53706
Phone: (608) 262-1416

WYOMING

School of Pharmacy
University of Wyoming
P.O. Box 3375
Laramie, WY 82071-3375
Phone: (307) 766-6120

Chapter 3

Pharmacy School: What You Can Expect

Introduction

You've made one of the most important decisions in your life. You've enrolled in pharmacy school.

What can you expect? Will the courses be a lot harder than those of your prepharmacy years? Will you be able to juggle your studies with a part-time job or with family responsibilities? What will your fellow students be like? How accessible will faculty be?

Will you make it?

These questions face you and more than 8,000 other students who enter pharmacy school each year. To get some trustworthy opinions, let's return to the pharmacy students featured at the beginning of Chapter 2. This time, they were asked two questions: What do you like best and least about pharmacy school? What surprised you?

• Tim admitted that the "intensity" of the studies surprised him. As his studies progressed, he felt a need for more up-to-date information on career options. (That's because this *Companion* had not yet been published!)

• Melissa was bothered by public misperceptions of pharmacists. "Now I know more than ever," she exclaimed, "that we don't just 'count and pour.'" She's intent on preparing for a career in a nontraditional setting.

• Eager to apply what he'd learned, Jim M. wished that experiential opportunities were available earlier in the course of study. Given the number of new careers opening up in pharmacy, he believed that students should be able to take more elective courses.

29

- Jim B. said that pharmacy school was "culture shock." He came from a small college. He found it hard to adjust to the independence and lack of opportunity for team study at his large pharmacy school.

- Todd was pleased at the amount of input he could give to creating his schedule and selecting courses.

- Amy D. termed her course in medicinal chemistry a "nightmare." She expressed a preference for more experiential training as well as for more involvement with the other schools of health professions on her campus.

- Darrell praised courses that use the problem-based learning approach. He thinks it's far superior to the traditional lecture methods that he'd come to expect in science.

- Charlotte was delighted that her school offered the opportunity to study anatomy and physiology with a computer program. It allows self-paced learning.

- Amy W. also liked the problem-based learning approach. She felt that being able to see patient charts early in her course of study gave her a good introduction to the real meaning of pharmaceutical care. The more that course work is coordinated, the better. When what you've struggled to learn in medicinal chemistry is followed up in pharmacology, and then in therapeutics, the whole system begins to make sense!

- Marci was enthusiastic about the opportunities to get involved in student association work because she felt they linked her directly with national affairs. Now in her fourth year, she expressed a desire that the curriculum introduce practice information earlier.

The Pharmacy Curriculum

As these students' observations indicate, when you enroll in pharmacy school, you've got five or six years of hard work ahead. The curriculum is intense. It's best to go into it with some clear expectations.

The next part of this chapter gives you an idea of what you can look forward to during your undergraduate years. The last part takes a giant leap ahead and provides a brief introduction to graduate study in pharmacy. Graduate studies, as well as residencies and fellowships (see Chapter 6), are all options for pharmacy graduates who wish to further their education and training. This chapter also includes a comprehensive table listing scholarships, internships, and other award programs available to pharmacy students and graduates.

Classroom and Laboratory Course Work

Don't expect to see a patient (or even a patient chart) during your first week or so of school. In the first year, you'll probably be taking courses such as communications, pharmacy and health care, pharmacy mathematics, anatomy and physiology, introductory pharmacy laboratory, medical terminology, biochemistry, microbiology, instrumental analysis, and health assessment.

Each year, you will be exposed to more practice-specific work. You will take courses in biopharmaceutics, pharmacology, pharmacokinetics, physical pharmacy and pharmaceutics, drug information, pathophysiology and therapeutics, pharmacy law, and dosage form design.

Problem-oriented learning is becoming popular on many campuses today. In comparison with the traditional didactic (lecture-based) learning method, the problem-based approach involves real-life patient scenarios. Students are challenged to apply what they've learned in previous courses to solve these patient problems. Problem-oriented learning is active rather than passive. For this reason, many pharmacy students find it particularly exciting.

Externships, Internships, and Clerkships

The classroom and laboratory work of your early years in pharmacy school prepare you to begin to gain practical experience in community and health-system settings. These experiences are called externships, internships, and clerkships. You must complete practical experience in at least two of these three categories before you can sit for your licensure examination (see Chapter 7).

Externships are structured general pharmacy experiences designed to introduce the student to many segments of pharmacy practice. The externship usually lasts between six and eight weeks. The student does not receive financial compensation for his or her work but does receive academic credit.

Clerkships (often called rotations) are structured training periods that expose the student to practice in a specific area. Clerkships are offered, for example, in nursing home consulting, toxicology, and infectious diseases. Each clerkship lasts for four to six weeks. A student may have several clerkship experiences. Like externships, clerkships offer academic credit but no pay.

Internships carry no academic credit but do provide financial reimbursement. Most states require completion of a certain number of internship hours (the minimum is usually 1,500) before allowing a candidate to sit for the licensing examination. Internship hours may be acquired before and after graduation. They are offered not only in community pharmacies and hospitals but also in managed care, government institutions, and other sites. Information on some internships, research experiences, and fellowships offered by national organizations appears in Appendix B at the end of the chapter.

Scholarships

Financial assistance and scholarships for pharmacy students are available from a number of sources, including the federal government, state governments, private foundations, and professional and civic groups.

Contact your dean's office for information. You may also want to consult scholarship directories. Undergraduate scholarships are included in Appendix B.

Making a Pledge

When you enter pharmacy school, you assume responsibility for maintaining the highest degree of conduct in all aspects of your educational and professional endeavors. The Pharmacy Student's Pledge of Professionalism (see sidebar, next page), developed by the American Pharmaceutical Association Academy of Students of Pharmacy and the American Association of Colleges of Pharmacy Council of Deans Task Force on Professionalism, summarizes the standards to which pharmacy students aspire.

Read it over thoughtfully. If someone at your school has not already done so, you may want to use it as the basis for creating a pledge for students at your own college or school.

Graduate Programs in Pharmacy

If you are interested in a position of leadership in a universi-

Pharmacy Student's Pledge of Professionalism

As a student of pharmacy, I believe there is a need to build and reinforce a professional identity founded on integrity, ethical behavior, and honor. This development, a vital process in my education, will help to ensure that I am true to the professional relationship I establish between myself and society as I become a member of the pharmacy community. Integrity will be an essential part of my everyday life and I will pursue all academic and professional endeavors with honesty and commitment to service.

To accomplish this goal of professional development, as a student of pharmacy I will:

A. DEVELOP a sense of loyalty and duty to the profession by contributing to the well-being of others and by enthusiastically accepting the responsibility and accountability for membership in the profession.

B. FOSTER professional competency through life-long learning. I will strive for high ideals, teamwork, and unity within the profession in order to provide optimal patient care.

C. SUPPORT my colleagues by actively encouraging personal commitment to the Oath of a Pharmacist and the Code of Ethics for Pharmacists as set forth by the profession.

D. DEDICATE my life and practice to excellence. This will require an ongoing reassessment of personal and professional values.

E. MAINTAIN the highest ideals and professional attributes to ensure and facilitate the covenantal relationship required of the pharmaceutical care giver.

The profession of pharmacy is one that demands adherence to a set of ethical principles. These high ideals are necessary to ensure the quality of care extended to the patients I serve. As a student of pharmacy, I believe this does not start with graduation; rather it begins with my membership in this professional college community. Therefore, I will strive to uphold this pledge as I advance toward full membership in the profession.

I voluntarily make this pledge of professionalism.

Developed and adopted by the American Pharmaceutical Association Academy of Students of Pharmacy/American Association of Colleges of Pharmacy Council of Deans Task Force on Professionalism, June 26, 1994. This pledge is offered as a model for adaptation by each school and college of pharmacy's faculty and students for use and reference in the professionalization of developing members of the pharmacy profession.

Adapted from the University of Illinois College of Pharmacy's Pledge of Professionalism (1993).

---

ty, the pharmaceutical industry, or the federal government, you may wish to earn a postgraduate degree. Such a degree will enable you to engage in basic research in the area of your choice and contribute to the knowledge base in pharmacy and medicine, teach, design and develop new drug products, and manage scientific projects in your field of study.

Successful graduate students tend to be highly motivated, flexible, committed, creative, and well organized. They need to be bright, but they needn't be a genius. Most programs require a minimum 3.0 grade point average and solid scores on the Graduate Record Examination.

Research experience is a bonus. To get it, take advantage of research electives during your undergraduate years. Do a summer internship with a pharmaceutical company. Talk with faculty members in an area of science that interests you. Many will have some substantive work that you can perform.

A list of graduate programs offered by schools and colleges of pharmacy in 1996-97 appears in Appendix C. Many fields of study offer both a master's degree and a doctor of philosophy degree.

Major fields of study are as follows:

Medicinal Chemistry. Design and synthesis of chemicals for use in the treatment of disease.

Pharmaceutical Sciences. Broad area encompasses both traditional laboratory work (making ointments, lotions, etc.) and clinical study. The basis for all clinical study.

Pharmacology. Study of the action of medicines on the body. Deals with designing different forms of medication (e.g., liquid, injectable, suspension, tablet, capsule) for use in humans and animals.

Pharmacognosy. Study of the use of natural plant or animal substances as a source of medicinal chemicals. How to obtain, purify, study, and use these substances in humans and animals.

Pharmaceutics. Designing, fabricating, and evaluating drug dosage forms. Development of drug delivery devices to optimize the effects of drugs in the body.

Pharmacokinetics. What happens to a drug after it enters a biologic system. Drug absorption, distribution, metabolism, and excretion and how these functions differ among populations.

Pharmacy Practice. The practical aspects of providing pharmaceutical care. Consolidates knowledge gained in other disciplines and teaches the student how to apply it to a specific patient problem. A related course in therapeutics deals with applying pharmacology to the treatment of diseases in humans.

Social and Administrative Sciences. Human behavior as it relates to how and why individuals take medications (social sciences). Application of practices and principles of business and law to pharmacy practice (administrative sciences).

Toxicology. The negative effects of medicinal agents on humans and animals. One application of this specialty is working in a poison control center; another is designing research to identify safe drug dosages.

Print Resources

Here are some print resources that you may find helpful during your undergraduate and graduate education in pharmacy.

APhA Print Resources

The following print resources are available from APhA. Discounts are available for student members. Call 1-800-878-0729 to place an order or make an inquiry.

- Handbook of Nonprescription Drugs
- Drug Information Handbook
- Patient Counseling Handbook
- Pocket Guide to Evaluations of Drug Interactions
- The One-Minute Counselor
- APhA Guide to Drug Treatment Protocols
- Comprehensive Pharmacy Review
- Pharmacy Drug Cards
- Stedman's Medical Dictionary
- Strauss's Federal Drug Laws and Examination Review
- Physical Assessment: A Guide for Evaluating Drug Therapy
- Handbook of Basic Pharmacokinetics
- Principles of Drug Information and Scientific Literature Evaluation
- Points of Light: A Guide for

33

Assisting Chemically Dependent Health Professional Students.

Other Print Resources

Glaxo Pathway Evaluation Program

Offers pharmacy students an organized approach to matching personal strengths and interests with the many career opportunities for pharmacists.

Glaxo Wellcome Explorer Monographs

Offers information about nonpractitioner pharmacist career options. (Note: There are facilitators for these two Glaxo programs at each college or school of pharmacy.)

Pharmacy School Admission Requirements

Contains information and names of contacts for all colleges and schools of pharmacy in the United States. Lists post-B.S. Pharm.D. programs, dual-degree programs, and characteristics of nontraditional Pharm.D. programs. Updated annually. $28. Available from the American Association of Colleges of Pharmacy at (703) 739-2330.

A Graduate Degree in the Pharmaceutical Sciences

Describes the options for graduate study in the pharmaceutical sciences. $20. Available from the American Association of Colleges of Pharmacy at (703) 739-2330.

Graduate School and You: A Guide for Prospective Graduate Students

Includes information on preparing for graduate school, selecting a school, sources of financial aid, and other issues. Published by the Educational Testing Service. For information, call (609) 683-2002.

"Opportunities in Independent Pharmacy"

Brochure describing the practice of independent pharmacy. Available from the National Community Pharmacists Association at (703) 683-8200.

Videotapes

"The Choice Is Yours: Pharmacy Careers in Organized Health-Care Settings"

A 15-minute tape describing pharmacy careers in health care systems. $100. Available from the American Society of Health-System Pharmacists. Call (301) 657-3000.

"The Invisible Ingredient"

A 15-minute video describing the role of the hospital pharmacist in patient care. $100. Available from the American Society of Health-System Pharmacists. Call (301) 657-3000.

"I Chose Industry"

A 10-minute video that describes a wide variety of opportunities in the pharmaceutical industry. Available from the Pharmaceutical Research and Manufacturers of America. Call (202) 835-3400.

"Pharmacy Entrepreneurs: A Closer Look"

A 17-minute video that highlights the careers of seven independent pharmacy practitioners. Available from the National Community Pharmacists Association at (703) 683-8200.

Internet Addresses

Check out the following sites on the World Wide Web. A wealth of information is at your fingertips!

Begin all addresses with "http://".

General Information
American Pharmaceutical Association
(www.aphanet.org)

Information about the association and its products and services, updates on legislative and regulatory issues of interest to pharmacists, and serious drug recall alerts. Includes special content area for students.

PharmWeb
(www.pharmweb.com)
Provides a link to national and international pharmacy sites. Has newsgroups, conferences, publications, pharmacy school lists. A good place to begin your search.

Auburn University Pharmacy Care Systems Home Page
(www.auburn.edu/pcs.html)
Information on innovative pharmacy practitioners, pharmacy automation systems, and facility design; reviews pharmacy software; much more.

Virtual Library for Pharmacy
(www/cpb/uokhsc.edu/ pharmacy/pharmint/html)
Many links to pharmacy sites on the Web.

Pharm Information Network
(www.pharminfo.com)
Links to other pharmacy, drug information, and health-related sites. Publications, job lists, conferences, and software developments.

Information on Specific Topics

International Pharmacy
(www.bton.ac.uk/pharmacy/ links.html)
Operated by the Department of Pharmacy, University of Brighton, United Kingdom.

Internet Drug Index
(www.rxlist.com)
Information about medications.

Pharmacokinetics
(www.cpb.uokhsc.edu/pkin/ pkin.html)

Pharmacokinetics, Pharmacodynamics, and Biopharmaceutics Home Page
(griffin.vcu.edu/~gkrishna/ PK/pk.html)

Insurance for Students, Inc.
(www.ins-for-students.com)

Women's Health
(www.ivf.com)

Federal Government Web Sites

The following Web sites are operated by the United States government. They may provide helpful information for a research or class project. The agencies are listed in alphabetical order.

- Agency for Health Care Policy and Research: www.ahcpr.gov

- Centers for Disease Control and Prevention: www.cdc.gov

- Consumer Health Information: odphp2.osophs.dhhs.gov/consumer.htm

- Consumer Product Safety Commission: www.cpsc.gov

- Environmental Protection Agency: www.epa.gov

- Food and Drug Administration: www.fda.gov

- Health Care Financing Administration: www.hcfa.gov

- Healthy People 2000: odphp.osophs.dhhs.gov/pubs/hp2000

- Indian Health Service: www.tucson.ihs.gov

- National Cancer Institute: cancernet.nci.nih.gov

- National Clearinghouse for Alcohol and Drug Information: www.health.org

- National Health Information Center: nhic-nt.health.org

- National Institute of Mental Health: www.nami.org

- National Institutes of Health: www.nih.gov

- Occupational Safety and Health Administration: www.osha.gov

- Office of Disease Prevention and Health Promotion: odphp.osophs.dhhs.gov

Appendix B

Scholarships, Loans, Awards, Grants, Internships, and Research Experiences

Scholarships

Title	Eligibility/Description	Award	Annual Deadline	Information
AAPS-AFPE Gateway Scholarships	Must be enrolled in the last three years of 1) a B.S. or Pharm.D. program in an accredited college of pharmacy or 2) a baccalaureate degree program in a related field of scientific study and show interest in and potential for a career in any of the pharmaceutical sciences. U.S. citizenship or permanent residence status is not required. Four awards given.	$9,250	December 1	AAPS-AFPE Gateway Scholarship Program One Church Street, Suite 202 Rockville, MD 20850 (301) 738-2160 FAX (301) 738-2161
AFPE-AACP First Year Graduate Student Scholarships	Must have participated in AACP Research Participation Program or Merck Research Scholar Program for Professional Pharmacy Students, and show proof of acceptance into PhD program in pharmaceutical discipline; U.S. citizen or permanent resident. Twelve awards given.	$5,000	May 1	AFPE Foundation (Address and Phone #'s same as above)
AFPE-Merck, AFPE-Sandoz, AFPE-Schein Gateway Scholarships	Must be enrolled in the last three years of a B.S. or Pharm.D. program and planning to pursue the Ph.D. in a college of pharmacy graduate program. Three awards given.	$9,250	December 1	AFPE Gateway Scholarship Program (Address and Phone #'s same as above)
AFPE Glaxo Wellcome First Year Graduate Studies Scholarship Program	Students in final year of B.S. or Pharm.D. program in pharmacy school; planning to pursue graduate or professional degree (not Pharm.D.) that will provide background for pharmaceutical industry career. Eight awards given.	$5,000	May 1	AFPE Foundation (Address and Phone #'s same as above)
AFPE-Sandoz, AFPE-SmithKline Beecham First Year Graduate Scholarships	Final year undergraduates or recent graduates planning to pursue Ph.D. in a pharmaceutical discipline in a pharmacy college. Must be U.S. citizen or permanent resident. Four awards given.	$5,000	May 1	AFPE Foundation (Address and Phone #'s same as above) or pharmacy dean's office
APhA/3M Partners for a Healthy Community Scholarships	Presented to one pharmacy student in each region who provides leadership and service in the delivery of patient education programs. Available to full-time pharmacy students who are members of APhA-ASP. Eight awards given.	$500	November 1	APhA 2215 Constitution Avenue, NW Washington, DC 20037 (202) 628-4410
Kappa Epsilon-AFPE Nellie Wakeman Scholarship	Member in good standing of Kappa Epsilon who has completed one quarter/semester of advanced studies in pharmaceutical sciences; need for financial assistance considered.	$4,000	May 1	KE Executive Office P.O. Box 870393 Stone Mountain, GA 33087 (404) 806-1312
Phi Lambda Sigma-Glaxo-AFPE First Year Graduate Scholarship	Must be in final year of a pharmacy B.S. or Pharm.D. program, and be a member of Phi Lambda Sigma. Must be U.S. citizen or have permanent residence status.	$7,500	January 15	AFPE Foundation One Church Street, Suite 202 Rockville, MD 20850 (301) 738-2160 FAX (301) 738-2161
Rho Chi-AFPE First Year Graduate Scholarship	Must be in final year of a pharmacy B.S. or Pharm.D. program, and be a member of Rho Chi. Must be U.S. citizen or have permanent residence status.	$7,500	January 15	AFPE Foundation (Address and Phone #'s same as above)
NACDS-AFPE Gateway Undergraduate Research Scholarship	Student enrolled in the last three years of B.S. or Pharm.D. program in a college of pharmacy. U.S. citizenship or permanent resident status is required.	$4,250	January 25	AFPE (Address and Phone #'s same as above)
NCPA Foundation Presidential Scholarships	NCPA student members enrolled full time in accredited U.S. pharmacy school. Award based on academic achievement/leadership qualities. Number of awards varies.	$2,000	Early March	NCPA Foundation 205 Daingerfield Road Alexandria, VA 22314 (703) 683-8200

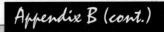

Appendix B (cont.)

Loans

Title	Eligibility/Description	Award	Annual Deadline	Information
Irene Parks Student Loan Fund (APhA Auxiliary)	Applicant must be in last two years of pharmacy program.	Up to $500	October 22	Ann Gagnon 13833 Hadley Overland Park, KS 66213
NCPA Foundation Student Loan Program	NCPA student member enrolled in final 2¼ years of first professional degree; U.S. citizen; minimum 2.5 GPA, cumulative and term prior to loan request.	$1,500 maximum per semester depending on tuition/fees	July 12 for fall term; November 15 for winter or spring term	NCPA Foundation 205 Daingerfield Road Alexandria, VA 22314 (703) 683-8200
U.S. Dept. of Health & Human Services Health Education and Assistance Loans (HEAL)	U.S. citizens or permanent residents; eligible graduate students in schools of pharmacy; full-time student in good standing at eligible HEAL school; must have satisfactorily completed three years training toward pharmacy degree.	$12,500 and $20,000	Unspecified	U.S. Dept. of HHS Division of Student Assistance HEAL 5600 Fishers Lane, Room 8-37 Rockville, MD 20857-0000
U.S. Dept. of Health & Human Services Health Professional Student Loans (HPSL)	U.S. citizen or permanent resident; financial need.	Unspecified	Set by school	U.S. Dept. of HHS Division of Student Assistance HPSL 5600 Fishers Lane, Room 834 Rockville, MD 20857-0000
U.S. Dept. of Health & Human Services Loans for Disadvantaged Students (LDS)	Enrolled full time in approved health professions school; financial need; minority or disadvantaged background.	Unspecified	Set by school	U.S. Dept. of HHS Division of Student Assistance LDS 5600 Fishers Lane Rockville, MD 20857-0000

Awards

Title	Eligibility/Description	Award	Annual Deadline	Information
APhA Student Leadership Award (supported by Procter & Gamble Health Care)	APhA-ASP member entering next-to-last professional year at accredited pharmacy school; accumulated GPA 2.75 or above. Elected national APhA-ASP officers not eligible.	$500	October 15	APhA-ASP chapter president or chapter advisor at each school
ASHP Research and Education Foundation Student Research Award	Full-time pharmacy students in B.S., M.S., or Pharm.D. program. Award for published or unpublished paper on subject relevant to health-system pharmacy practice.	$1000 + $700 travel to ASHP Midyear Clinical Meeting	May 15	ASHP Research and Education Foundation 7272 Wisconsin Avenue Bethesda, MD 20814 (301) 657-3000, ext 1351
NCPA Student Achievement Award	Students at every U.S. college of pharmacy who (1) have at least one year left, (2) are interested in a career in one of the many unique practice settings available in independent pharmacy, and (3) have the entrepreneurial spirit that these individuals foster en route to achieving their goals.	$200 + a recognition plaque	Rolling	School awards committee; or NCPA Student Affairs 205 Daingerfield Road Alexandria, VA 22314 (703) 683-8200

Appendix B (cont.)

Grants

Title	Eligibility/Description	Award	Annual Deadline	Information
ASHP Research and Education Foundation New Pharmacy Practice Researchers Grants	Pharmacists within five years of graduation. Seed money for new pharmacy investigators; research topics are designated each year; applicants must submit proposal and budget.	Up to $6,000	June 1	ASHP Research and Education Foundation 7272 Wisconsin Avenue Bethesda, MD 20814 (301) 657-3000, ext. 1351
PDA Faculty Development Grant	Individuals beginning their career at the faculty level in fields pertinent to parenteral drugs such as pharmacy, pharmacology, and manufacturing.	$15,000	April 1	PDA, Inc. 7500 Old Georgetown Road, Suite 620 Bethesda, MD 20814 (301) 986-0293

Internships

Title	Eligibility/Description	Award	Annual Deadline	Information
AACP Elective Experiential Rotation	Enrolled in professional pharmacy degree programs or graduate degree programs in the pharmaceutical sciences. Provides experiences in national pharmacy association activities and operations.	Housing: subject to availability	Rolling: most selections made spring of preceding academic year	AACP 1426 Prince Street Alexandria, VA 22314 (703) 739-2330
Amgen Summer Internship Program	Undergraduate students planning careers in a scientific discipline who have completed the sophomore year. 10 weeks, May-September, in research environment. Sixty or more awards given.	Stipend	March 15	Laurie Dozier Amgen, Inc. 1840 DeHavilland Drive Thousand Oaks, CA 91320 (805) 447-4354
APhA-ASP Experiential Externship Program	An elective rotation in national association management available to students pursuing an entry-level degree in pharmacy. The rotation is structured to provide experiences in national association activities.	N/A	Rolling	APhA-ASP 2215 Constitution Ave., NW Washington, DC 20037 (202) 429-7595
APhA-ASP Industry Internship Program	Full time pharmacy students with graduation dates prior to 5/2000. Must be APhA-ASP members. Provides general, clinical, and research experiences in the pharmaceutical industry.	Stipend set by host	Last working day in November	APhA, Industry Internship Program 2215 Constitution Ave, NW Washington DC 20037 (202) 628-4410
APhA-ASP Summer Internship	Any B.S. or Pharm.D. undergraduate who has completed at least one professional year. Ten weeks; emphasis on pharmacy affairs.	Stipend	March 1	APhA-ASP 2215 Constitution Ave., NW Washington, DC 20037 (202) 628-4410
ASHP Summer Internship	Any B.S. or Pharm.D. undergraduate who has completed at least one professional year. Ten weeks; emphasis on membership services, particularly student affairs.	Stipend	February 1	ASHP 7272 Wisconsin Avenue Bethesda, MD 20814 (301) 657-3000
Consumer Health Information Corporation Summer Intern Program	Full-time pharmacy student entering final year of undergraduate degree or completed undergraduate degree and enrolled in Pharm.D. program. 10-12 weeks. Work on current projects developing patient education programs.	Stipend	March 1	Jill Devrick, Executive Assistant Consumer Health Information Corporation 8300 Greensboro Drive, Suite 1220 McLean, VA 22102 (703) 734-0650

Appendix B (cont.)

Title	Eligibility/Description	Award	Annual Deadline	Information
George P. Provost Editorial Internship	Any pharmacy school graduate. Six months at ASHP headquarters; focus on pharmaceutical writing, editing, publishing.	Stipend	February 1	Chairman, Editorial Internship Selection Committee ASHP 7272 Wisconsin Avenue Bethesda, MD 20814 (301) 657-3000, ext. 1251
NACDS Summer Internship Program	Full-time pharmacy student in good academic standing who has completed the first year of pharmacy school. Six- to nine-week program.	Stipend	Postmarked by March 14	Sandra Kay Jung, Manager of Professional Services and Programs NACDS Pharmacy Affairs Department P.O. Box 1417-D49 Alexandria, VA 22313-1480 (703) 549-3001
NCPA Summer Intern Program	Full-time pharmacy student entering final year of first professional degree; minimum cumulative GPA of 2.5. 10-week experiential program.	N/A	Rolling	NCPA 205 Daingerfield Road Alexandria, VA 22314 (703) 683-8200
Paul G. Cano Legislative Internship Program	Full-time pharmacy students entering the final year of an accredited program in fall. Eight weeks (June-August); focus on government affairs.	Stipend and travel expenses	March 15	Leigh Davitan ASCP 1321 Duke Street Alexandria, VA 22314 (703) 739-1300
AMCP/Parke-Davis Managed Care Pharmacy Summer Internship Program	Full-time enrollment in accredited school of pharmacy, B.S. or Pharm.D. 10-12 weeks. May-August 1997; includes activities in managed care practice sites, professional association, industry.	Stipend	March 15	Beth Levine or Jennifer Lucas Medication Education Systems, Inc. (800) 229-9840 (215) 665-1060
Public Health Service Commissioned Officer Student Training and Extern Program (COSTEP)	Completion of at least two years of approved pharmacy program, expect to return the next semester after internship. Serve as junior assistant health service officer at one of five PHS agencies.	Paid assignment	Oct 1 for Jan-Apr Dec 1 for May-Aug May 1 for Sept-Dec	COSTEP Division of Commissioned Personnel Parklawn Bldg., Room 435 5600 Fishers Lane Rockville, MD 20857
United States Pharmacopeia (USP) Summer Internship Program	Pharmacy students in their final two professional years, or recent graduates. 12 weeks; specific projects in Division of Information Development, Practitioners Reporting Network, Professional and Public Affairs.	$6,000	March 15	USP Dept. of Professional and Public Affairs 12601 Twinbrook Parkway Rockville, MD 20852 (301) 816-8283

Research Experiences

Title	Eligibility/Description	Award	Annual Deadline	Information
AACP/Merck Research Scholar Program for Professional Students in Pharmacy	Pharmacy students who completed at least one professional year. Pharmaceutical sciences research experience for students considering graduate studies in the pharmaceutical sciences. Must present results at AACP's Annual Meeting.	$6,000 stipend for full calendar year; $1,000 for research supplies to school	January 24	AACP 1426 Prince Street Alexandria, VA 22314 (703) 739-2330 or contact dean's office

Source: Interorganizational Council on Student Affairs, Interorganizational Financial and Experiential Information Document, July 18, 1996.

Appendix C

U.S. Graduate Programs in Pharmacy, 1996–97

School or College	Type of Program	Degree(s) Offered
Auburn	Pharmacal Sciences	MS PhD
	Pharmacy Care Systems	MS PhD
Arizona	Medicinal Chemistry/Natural Products	MS PhD
	Pharmaceutical Economics	MS PhD
	Pharmaceutics	MS PhD
	Pharmacology/Toxicology	MS PhD
Arkansas	Pharmaceutical Sciences	MS
California- San Francisco	Pharmaceutical Chemistry	PhD
University of the Pacific	Pharmaceutical Sciences	MS PhD
Southern California	Molecular Pharmacology and Toxicology	MS PhD
	Pharmaceutical Economics & Policy	MS PhD
	Pharmaceutical Sciences	MS PhD
Colorado	Pharmaceutical Sciences	MS PhD
	Toxicology	PhD
Connecticut	Medicinal & Natural Products Chemistry	MS PhD
	Pharmaceutics	MS PhD
	Pharmacology and Toxicology	MS PhD
Florida A & M	Pharmaceutical Sciences	MS PhD
Florida	Pharmaceutical Sciences	MS PhD
Mercer	Pharmaceutical Sciences	PhD
	Pharmacy Administration	MS
Georgia	Medicinal Chemistry	MS PhD
	Pharmaceutics	MS PhD
	Pharmacology and Toxicology	MS PhD
	Pharmacy Care Administration	MS PhD
Idaho State	Pharmaceutical Sciences	MS PhD
Illinois at Chicago	Medicinal Chemistry	MS PhD
	Pharmaceutics	MS PhD
	Pharmacodynamics	MS PhD
	Pharmacognosy	MS PhD
	Pharmacy Administration	MS PhD
Butler	Pharmaceutical Sciences	MS
Purdue	Health Sciences	MS
	Industrial and Physical Chemistry	PhD
	Medicinal Chemistry and Molecular Pharmacology	MS PhD
	Pharmacy Practice	MS PhD

School or College	Type of Program	Degree(s) Offered
Iowa	Clinical and Administrative Pharmacy	MS PhD
	Medicinal and Natural Products Chemistry	MS PhD
	Pharmaceutics	MS PhD
Kansas	Health Services Administration	MS
	Hospital Pharmacy	MS
	Medicinal Chemistry	MS PhD
	Pharmaceutical Chemistry	MS PhD
	Pharmacology and Toxicology	MS PhD
Kentucky	Pharmaceutical Sciences	MS PhD
NE Louisiana	Pharmaceutical Sciences/Pharmacy	MS PhD
Maryland	Pharmaceutical Sciences	MS PhD
	Pharmacy Administration	MS PhD
Massachusetts	Analytical Medicinal Chemistry	MS PhD
	Cosmetic Science	MS PhD
	Organic or Medicinal Chemistry	MS PhD
	Pharmaceutics/Industrial Pharmacy	MS PhD
	Pharmacology	MS PhD
Northeastern	Biomedical Sciences	MS PhD
	Medical Laboratory Science	MS PhD
	Medicinal Chemistry	MS PhD
	Pharmaceutics	MS PhD
	Pharmacology	MS PhD
	Toxicology	MS PhD
Michigan	Pharmaceutical Chemistry	MS PhD
	Pharmacy	MS PhD
	Medicinal Chemistry/Pharmacognosy	MS PhD
	Pharmaceutics	MS PhD
Wayne State	Health Systems Pharmacy Management	MS
	Pharmacy Science	MS PhD
Minnesota	Hospital Pharmacy	MS
	Medicinal Chemistry	MS PhD
	Pharmaceutics	MS PhD
	Social and Administrative Pharmacy	MS PhD
Mississippi	Medicinal Chemistry	MS PhD
	Pharmaceutics	MS PhD
	Pharmacognosy	MS PhD
	Pharmacology	MS PhD
	Pharmacy Administration	MS PhD

41

Appendix C (cont.)

School or College	Type of Program	Degree(s) Offered
St. Louis	Pharmacy Administration	MS
Missouri	Pharmaceutical Sciences	MS PhD
	Pharmacology	MS PhD
Montana	Pharmacy	MS
Nebraska	Pharmaceutical Sciences	MS PhD
Rutgers	Pharmaceutical Sciences	MS PhD
	Toxicology	MS PhD
New Mexico	Hospital Pharmacy	MS
	Pharmacy Administration	MS PhD
	Radiopharmacy	MS
	Toxicology	MS PhD
Arnold & Marie Schwartz	Cosmetic Science	MS
	Drug Information and Communication	MS
	Drug Regulatory Affairs	MS
	Hospital Pharmacy Administration	MS
	Industrial Pharmacy	MS
	Pharmaceutical and Health Care Marketing Administration	MS
	Pharmaceutics	PhD
	Pharmacology/Toxicology	MS
	Pharmacotherapeutics	MS
St. John's	Drug Information Specialist	MS
	Medical Technology	MS
	Pharmaceutical Sciences	MS PhD
	Pharmacy Administration	MS
	Toxicology	MS
Buffalo	Biochemical Pharmacology	MS PhD
	Medicinal Chemistry	MS PhD
	Pharmaceutics	MS PhD
North Carolina	Medicinal Chemistry	MS PhD
	Pharmaceutical Policy & Evaluative Sciences	MS
	Pharmaceutics	MS PhD
North Dakota State	Pharmaceutical Sciences	MS PhD
Ohio State	Hospital Pharmacy	MS
	Medicinal Chemistry and Pharmacognosy	MS PhD
	Pharmacy Administration	MS PhD
	Pharmaceutics and Pharmaceutical Chemistry	MS PhD
	Pharmacology	MS PhD
Cincinnati	Pharmaceutical Sciences	MS PhD
Toledo	Medicinal and Biological Chemistry	MS PhD
	Pharmaceutical Sciences	MS
Oklahoma	Pharmaceutical Sciences	MS PhD
Oregon State	Pharmaceutical Sciences	MS PhD
Mylan	Medicinal Chemistry	MS PhD

School or College	Type of Program	Degree(s) Offered
	Pharmaceutical Chemistry	MS PhD
	Pharmaceutics	MS PhD
	Pharmacology/Toxicology	MS PhD
Philadelphia	Chemistry	MS PhD
	Pharmaceutics	MS PhD
	Pharmacology/Toxicology	MS PhD
	Pharmacy Administration	MS PhD
Temple	Pharmaceutical Sciences	MS PhD
	Quality Assurance and Regulatory Affairs	MS
Pittsburgh	Clinical Sciences	PhD
	Pharmaceutical Sciences	PhD
Puerto Rico	Pharmacy	MS
Rhode Island	Pharmaceutical Sciences	PhD
	Pharmacology	MS
	Pharmacy Administration	MS
Medical U South Carolina	Pharmaceutical Sciences	PhD
South Carolina	Medicinal Chemistry	MS PhD
	Pharmaceutics	MS PhD
	Pharmacology	MS PhD
	Pharmacy Administration	MS PhD
Tennessee	Health Science Administration	MS PhD
	Pharmaceutical Sciences	PhD
Houston	Pharmaceutics	MS PhD
	Pharmacology	MS PhD
Texas at Austin	Medicinal Chemistry	MS PhD
	Pharmaceutics	MS PhD
	Pharmacy Administration	MS PhD
	Pharmacy/Toxicology	MS PhD
Utah	Medicinal Chemistry	MS PhD
	Pharmaceutics/Pharmaceutical Chemistry	MS PhD
	Pharmacology/Toxicology	MS PhD
Virginia Commonwealth	Medicinal Chemistry	MS PhD
	Pharmacy and Pharmaceutics	MS PhD
Washington	Medicinal Chemistry	MS PhD
	Pharmaceutical Sciences	MS PhD
	Pharmaceutics	MS PhD
Washington State	Health Policy and Administration	MS
	Pharmacology/Toxicology	MS PhD
West Virginia	Pharmaceutical Sciences	MS PhD
Wisconsin	Hospital Pharmacy	MS
	Pharmaceutical Sciences	MS PhD
	Social and Administrative Sciences	MS PhD

Source: American Association of Colleges of Pharmacy

Chapter 4

Involvement in the National Professional Society of Pharmacists

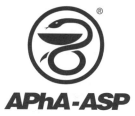

Introduction

The American Pharmaceutical Association's Academy of Students of Pharmacy (APhA-ASP) represents 18,000 pharmacy students. APhA-ASP has chapters at every school and college of pharmacy in the United States and Puerto Rico. The cost of a one-year active membership in the national association is only $25 (local chapter dues are extra). Even if you're a financially pressed student, it's bound to be among the best investments you'll ever make.

Why join a student pharmacy association? It's a great way to meet people. Membership grants you access to pharmacy practitioners at the state, regional, and national levels. It gives you a structured opportunity to meet other pharmacy students—those in your class and those above and below you. You'll be exposed to new ways of thinking, meet potential employers, and make friends. Many pharmacists have found that relationships born during their days as a member of APhA-ASP last a lifetime.

Membership also provides other benefits, such as a subscription to APhA's journal. You'll be able to attend APhA meetings at reduced student rates. While there, you'll attend special programs designed for students.

History of APhA–ASP

APhA-ASP was unofficially established in 1921, when students of the University of North Carolina petitioned the APhA Council to be recognized as an APhA student branch. Shortly thereafter, other schools of pharmacy began to form student branches.

Student participation grew steadily. In 1954, a formal student section was created, largely as a result of the efforts of the late Linwood F. Tice. Creation of the student section allowed students to send a delegate to the APhA House of Delegates. In 1969, APhA members approved new bylaws that created three Association subdivisions, one of which was the Student American Pharmaceutical Association (SAPhA).

Between 1969 and 1979, the number of student delegates in the APhA House of Delegates increased from 1 to 15. The number of student delegates rose to 28 in 1986 following passage of new APhA bylaws that created the APhA Academy of Students of Pharmacy and put students on equal footing with the other two APhA academies. In 1994, APhA's Academy of Students of Pharmacy marked its 25th anniversary as an official section of the association.

Governing Structure

The country is divided into eight regions, each of which elects its own regional officers (delegate, regional member-at-large, and Midyear Regional Meeting coordinator) at the APhA-ASP Midyear Regional Meetings each fall.

APhA-ASP is represented on the national level by a five-member Executive Committee consisting of a president, president-elect, two members-at-large, and the speaker of the APhA-ASP House of Delegates. National officers are elected each spring at the APhA Annual Meeting and Exposition. Each APhA-ASP chapter elects its own officers.

Mission of the APhA Academy of Students of Pharmacy

The mission of the APhA Academy of Students of Pharmacy is to prepare pharmacy students to be professionals who provide and promote pharmaceutical care.

The 1996-97 APhA-ASP Executive Committee outlined the following objectives to achieve the goals of the APhA Academy of Students of Pharmacy:

Goal 1 Promote the value of pharmaceutical care to the public.

Goal 2 Promote the development of professional attitudes and behaviors in pharmacy students.

Goal 3 Advance pharmaceutical education to reflect a greater emphasis on pharmaceutical care.

Goal 4 Promote interdisciplinary teamwork to foster professional relationships and increase the quality of patient care.

Goal 5 Position APhA–ASP as the unified voice for pharmacy students.

Goal 6 Increase pharmacy student involvement in the American Pharmaceutical Association.

Membership in APhA–ASP

Eligibility

Any pharmacy student is eligible for student membership in APhA-ASP. A student is defined as any individual regularly enrolled in either a prepharmacy or professional pharmacy practice degree program in a university or college holding membership in the American Association of Colleges of Pharmacy or accredited by the American Council on Pharmaceutical Education.

Membership Categories

There are two APhA-ASP membership categories.

Active student members must belong to an APhA-ASP chapter at one of the schools or colleges of pharmacy. They receive three APhA publications (*Journal of the American Pharmaceutical Association, Pharmacy Student*, and *Pharmacy Today*), discounts on APhA publications, and reduced registration for APhA meetings. They also have access to financial services (e.g., a credit card, liability insurance, life insurance). They can hold elective office in the association. Any prepharmacy student attending a university with an accredited pharmacy school can become an active member.

Associate student members are prepharmacy students who attend a college or university that does not have an accredited pharmacy school. Associate student members gain access to professional information and an opportunity to meet pharmacy students and practitioners who can help share information on their careers. They receive *Pharmacy Student* and *Pharmacy Today* and have access to discounts on APhA publications and reduced registration fees to professional meetings. They also have access to a variety of financial and professional services. Associate student members may not vote or hold office. They may join through the APhA national headquarters by calling (800) 237-APhA.

Dues

The annual dues for active student members are $25. Many chapters assess additional dues to fund local activities. Dues for associate student members are $45 per year. Students have the option of joining their state pharmacy association at the same time they join APhA-ASP.

Membership Year

The APhA-ASP membership year runs from November 1 through October 31. If students enroll before November 1, their benefits will begin immediately.

Member Benefits

Personal and Professional Growth

Through involvement in APhA's Academy of Students of Pharmacy, members have the opportunity to

- Develop skills they can't learn in a classroom.
- Learn how to organize people and resources.
- Participate in professional service projects.
- Motivate themselves and others.
- Turn ideas into results.

A Role in Shaping the Profession

The APhA House of Delegates, the association's official policy-making body, makes recommendations on issues affecting the profession and students. Twenty-eight students serve in the APhA House of Delegates. Any APhA-ASP member may submit proposals for consideration by the House of Delegates.

A Voice in Washington

APhA monitors legislative activity on issues that affect the future of APhA-ASP members, such as health care reform and student financial aid. APhA also represents pharmacy's interests before the U.S. Congress and federal regulatory agencies.

Leadership Opportunities

APhA-ASP gives members the opportunity to chair committees, serve as chapter officers, serve in the APhA-ASP House of Delegates, and become regional or national APhA-ASP officers. APhA provides opportunities for students to develop leadership skills that they can use in their community and their profession.

Chapter Activities

Membership in the local APhA-ASP chapter automatically provides students with membership in APhA at the national level. APhA-ASP chapters offer many opportunities for member involvement at the school and community levels. Chapter meetings, health fairs, socials, fund raising, elections, membership drives, and community education are among the activities in which members may participate.

Career Development

APhA-ASP provides many opportunities for students to explore their career options. A Career Expo, held during the APhA Annual Meeting and Exposition, offers students the opportunity to interview with companies from all over the United States. The Midyear Regional Meetings feature the APhA-ASP MRM PharmExpo. This exhibit gives pharmacy students the opportunity to meet representatives from the pharmaceutical industry and potential employers from various practice and educational settings.

International Membership

APhA-ASP is a member of the International Pharmaceutical Students' Federation (IPSF). Members of APhA-ASP are automatically members of IPSF. This gives them the opportunity to participate in the IPSF's international Student Exchange Program and attend the IPSF Annual Congress.

Academy Membership

When students join APhA, they automatically become members of the APhA-ASP. Upon graduation, membership in APhA continues. The graduate may become a New Practitioner active member and select an academy affiliation in the Academy of Pharmacy Practice and Management (APhA-APPM) or the Academy of Pharmaceutical Research and Science (APhA-APRS).

APhA–ASP Meetings

Midyear Regional Meetings, held each fall in eight cities across the country (see sidebar next page for 1997 schedule), provide information on career options, legislative issues affecting the profession, chapter development, and other topics of particular interest to students. At these meetings, chapter representatives elect regional APhA-ASP officers and propose topics for APhA-ASP resolution.

The APhA Annual Meeting and Exposition, held each March, provides APhA-ASP members the opportunity to participate in discussions on contemporary issues, elect APhA-ASP officers, enhance their career opportunities, and meet colleagues from across the nation and around the world. The 1998 APhA Annual Meeting will be held in Miami Beach, Florida, on March 21-25.

Awards Program

APhA-ASP members are eligible for consideration for national awards such as the APhA Stu-

1997 APhA-ASP MRMs

Region	Location	Dates
1	Buffalo, NY	October 31-November 1
2	Richmond, VA	October 24-26
3	Charleston, SC	October 17-19
4	Toledo, OH	October 24-26
5	Iowa City, IA	November 7-9
6	St. Louis, MO	October 17-19
7	Pocatello, ID	October 31-November 1
8	Los Angeles, CA	November 7-9

dent Leadership Award, the APhA-ASP Senior Recognition Award, and the APhA-ASP Mortar and Pestle Professionalism Award.

Subscriptions to APhA Publications

Journal of the American Pharmaceutical Association (JAPhA), APhA's official, peer-reviewed journal, has articles on drug therapy and diseases, news and analysis of trends in pharmacy practice and therapeutics, and original research. Information is presented in a practice-oriented format.

Pharmacy Today, APhA's monthly newspaper, covers all areas of practice, including student news. It contains clinical drug information, legislative/regulatory/legal news, opinion pieces, human interest stories, and APhA news.

Pharmacy Student, a magazine designed specifically for pharmacy student members, provides tips for succeeding in school, updates on legislation, and career information as well as news briefs on science, health, drugs, education, and APhA activities.

APhA-ASP chapters receive *Chapter Management*, a monthly publication designed to help chapter officers and advisers manage chapter activities more efficiently and provide improved membership services.

Discounts on APhA Publications

Members receive substantial discounts on APhA publications. To obtain a copy of the APhA publications catalog or to order any APhA publications, call (800) 878-0729.

Other Benefits

Other benefits available to student members include:

• Professional liability insurance
• Life insurance, automobile insurance
• Financial services (APhA-ASP Student MasterCard, Member-loan Program, Gold Savers Money Market Account, credit union services)
• Discounts on car rental and long-distance telephone.

APhA–ASP Activities

APhA-ASP has many national programs and activities that are of interest to pharmacy and prepharmacy students at any point in their educational career. For more information on any of these programs, contact APhA at (800) 237-APhA or visit the APhA web site at http://www.aphanet.org.

APhA/Merck Student Pharmacy Project Grants

Up to ten $2,000 grants are awarded each year to APhA-ASP chapters. All APhA-ASP chapters are eligible to participate in the APhA/Merck Pharmacy Project Grant program. Grants are awarded to provide funding and national recognition for projects that foster pharmacy association activities as a vital element of pharmacy education.

APhA–National Council of State Pharmacy Association Executives Executive Residency in Association Management

This residency is available to any graduate of an accredited pharmacy school, licensed or immediately eligible for licensure following graduation. The Executive Residency is a postgraduate training program conducted at APhA in Washington, D.C., and at a selected state pharmacy association headquarters. This one-year program provides a quality, multisite training experience to develop well-qualified pharmacists to assume management positions in pharmacy-related organizations at both the state and national levels.

APhA-ASP/USP National Patient Counseling Competition

The objective of the APhA-ASP/USP National Patient Counseling Competition is to encourage pharmacy students in their efforts to become better patient educators. The competition reflects the changes that have already occurred in pharmacy practice, promotes and encourages further professional development, and demonstrates to students that there is genuine commitment by faculty to the concept of professional growth through innovation.

APhA Academy of Students of Pharmacy Industry Internship Program

Preference for the APhA Academy of Students of Pharmacy Industry Internship Program is given to students who have completed at least one professional year. Each industry internship is designed to add to the student's overall knowledge of pharmacy, especially its industrial aspect. The internship will enhance the student's knowledge of the pharmaceutical industry and its role in pharmacy and medicine. It may also suggest industry-related career opportunities and pathways for interested students.

International Pharmaceutical Students' Federation Student Exchange Program

The IPSF Student Exchange Program provides pharmacy students the opportunity to learn about pharmacy in another country or host an international student in the United States. Over 40 countries participate in the exchange program.

APhA Pharmacy Recovery Network

The APhA Pharmacy Recovery Network (PRN) is an informal informational network for people who are planning, or are currently active in, state pharmacy recovery programs; state and national pharmaceutical association executives; state board of pharmacy personnel; pharmacy school students, faculty and administrators; leaders in firms and organizations that employ pharmacists; pharmacist-related employee assistance program personnel; and people who are concerned about alcoholism and other drug dependencies in their colleagues.

University of Utah School on Alcoholism and Other Drug Dependencies

The internationally recognized University of Utah School on Alcoholism and Other Drug Dependencies was founded in 1951. The program increases awareness of the health and social problems of alcoholism and other drug dependencies. These problems are presented in training sessions for both professional and lay personnel. The school provides students with the latest methods and techniques for working to prevent substance abuse and assist recovering persons during treatment and follow-up. Each year, the school attracts hundreds of experts on substance abuse and provides programming for over 1,200 participants.

APhA/3M Partners for a Healthy Community Scholarship

The APhA/3M Partners for a Healthy Community Scholarship Program is an individual scholarship program designed to recognize pharmacy students and pharmacy practitioners who develop and participate in patient education projects. Through this program, APhA and 3M Pharmaceuticals will present a $500 cash award in each of the eight APhA regions to one pharmacist and one pharmacy student who have demonstrated leadership and service in the delivery of patient education programs.

APhA Community Pharmacy Residency Programs

Applicants for these residency programs (listed in Chapter 6) must possess an entry-level pharmacy degree from an accredited college of pharmacy. The goal of the community pharmacy residency programs is to provide structured and advanced education and training for pharmacists whose ability, motivation, and career aspirations suggest potential for creative and innovative leadership in community pharmacy practice. Education and training will be concentrated in the following areas: (1) delivery of pharmaceutical care in administration and management, (2) control of drug distribution and drug use, (3) clinical services, (4) drug information services, (5) home health care, (6) long-term care, and (7) areas of special interest.

APhA-ASP Experiential Externship Program

APhA offers an elective rotation in national association management to students pursuing an entry-level degree in pharmacy. The rotation is structured to provide experiences in national association activities and operations, pharmacy practice issues, educational programming, state services, scientific affairs, student affairs, public relations, and project management. The rotation schedule is designed to be four weeks in duration and is available throughout the year.

APhA-ASP Summer Internship in Association Management

APhA offers several 12-week summer internships in national association management to students pursuing an entry-level degree in pharmacy. The internship is structured to provide experiences in national association activities and operations while focusing on one area of interest throughout the internship.

National Pharmacy Week

National Pharmacy Week provides an opportunity for students to get involved in promoting the profession at the local or state level. APhA's Pharmacy Week Planning Guide helps students plan to get the most out of this observance. Each APhA-ASP chapter president receives a complimentary copy. Additional guides are available by calling (800) 822-1923.

Chapter 5

The World of Pharmacy Organizations

Introduction

As a student, you'll probably derive most satisfaction from membership in a student pharmacy association such as the American Pharmaceutical Association Academy of Students of Pharmacy. Even at this stage in your career, however, it's important to know that there are many other pharmacy organizations that offer valuable membership benefits.

This chapter provides information about many of these organizations. Entries are grouped into four categories: state APhA associations; national pharmacy organizations that have student membership categories; organizations that have only institutional members; and other organizations. You'll find Internet addresses of these and other health organizations at the end of the chapter.

State APhA Associations

There are state APhA pharmacy associations in all 50 states. Although the size of these associations differs widely, the benefits they offer are much the same. Membership in a state association gives pharmacists a unified voice on issues that concern them. Many state associations engage in active legislative efforts. State associations also offer educational programs at which members can gain continuing-education units needed for relicensure.

State associations offer many benefits for student members. For example, many sponsor licensure examination review

51

courses as well as other educational programs. Some sponsor annual legislative days that give members the opportunity to visit their congressional representatives to discuss issues of concern. State associations sponsor mentoring programs that bring together experienced practitioners and students. Many offer job placement services. Some offer student scholarships.

Membership policies and student dues vary from state to state. For information, contact your state association (see Appendix D at end of chapter).

Organizations with Student Membership Categories

Academy of Managed Care Pharmacy
1650 King Street, Suite 402
Alexandria, VA 22314
(800) TAP-AMCP

National professional society dedicated to the concept and practice of pharmaceutical care in managed health care environments.

Student memberships are available to students and residents enrolled in an accredited college of pharmacy or a residency program. AMCP has student chapters at the University of Illinois at Chicago and the Philadelphia College of Pharmacy and Science; additional student chapters are being formed.

Upcoming AMCP meetings: October 30-November 3, 1997, Educational Conference, Seattle, WA; April 30-May 4, 1998, 10th Annual Meeting, Philadelphia, PA. Registration fee for student members is $35.

American Association of Colleges of Pharmacy
1426 Prince Street
Alexandria, VA 22314
(703) 739-2330

Works to advance pharmaceutical education, research, and service in accredited pharmacy schools. Promotes the exchange of information among educators. Members include schools and colleges of pharmacy and individual faculty and administrators. Publishes the *American Journal of Pharmaceutical Education* and *ACCP News*.

Associate memberships are offered to undergraduate and graduate pharmacy students.

American College of Apothecaries
P.O. Box 341266
Memphis, TN 38184
(901) 383-8119

Works to advance pharmacy practice and enhance the professionalism of pharmacy practitioners. Publishes various newsletters and *The Voice of the Pharmacist*.

Student members must have completed at least two years of prepharmacy school and be enrolled in a college of pharmacy.

Upcoming ACA meetings: September 10-14, 1997, Palm Beach, FL; August 26-30, 1998, Ontario, Canada. Registration fees are waived for student members.

American College of Clinical Pharmacy
3101 Broadway, Suite 380
Kansas City, MO 64111
(816) 531-2177

Dedicated to optimizing drug therapy outcomes by promoting excellence in clinical pharmacy practice, research, and education. Provides educational programs; establishes and maintains standards for pharmacotherapists and clinical pharmacy researchers. Publishes *ACCP Report* and *Pharmacotherapy*.

Reduced membership dues are offered to students, residents, and fellows. Student members receive discounted registration rates at ACCP meetings. Other student membership benefits include the opportunity to participate in a special abstract category at the ACCP Spring Forum, awards for papers, networking opportunities, and placement services for specialty residencies and research fellowships.

Upcoming ACCP meetings: November 9-12, 1997, Annual Meeting, Phoenix, AZ; April 5-8, 1998, Spring Practice and Research Forum, Palm Springs, CA.

American Institute of the
History of Pharmacy
425 North Charter Street
Madison, WI 53706
(608) 262-5378

Works to preserve the historical contributions of pharmacists and the industry. Conducts research; maintains library; offers information and educational services. Publishes *AIHP Notes*. Student membership available at reduced rate. Meets annually with APhA.

American Pharmaceutical
Association
2215 Constitution Avenue, NW
Washington, DC 20037
(800) 237-APhA

Promotes quality health care and rational drug therapy; works to protect the public health and assure the quality of drug products; promotes high professional standards; represents pharmacy's interests and lobbies for the profession on legislative issues. Publications include *Pharmacy Today, Journal of the American Pharmaceutical Association, Journal of Pharmaceutical Sciences, Pharmacy Student*, and *Academy Reporter*.

Has three academies: the APhA Academy of Pharmacy Practice and Management, the APhA Academy of Pharmaceutical Research and Science, and the APhA Academy of Students of Pharmacy (APhA–ASP). Each APhA member may join one academy. Each academy has sections that focus on a particular aspect of its scope of interest, and each academy member may join one section.

The APhA-ASP has more than 18,000 members. For information on student membership, see Chapter 4.

Upcoming APhA meetings: March 21-25, 1998, Annual Meeting and Exposition, Miami Beach, FL. See Chapter 4 for the dates and locations of the eight APhA-ASP 1997 Midyear Regional Meetings.

American Society of Consultant
Pharmacists
1321 Duke Street
Alexandria, VA 22314
(703) 739-1300

The national professional association representing pharmacists who provide medication-distribution and consultant services to patients in long-term care facilities.

Student dues are $40 annually. Student members receive all the benefits of active members except the right to vote and hold office.

Upcoming ASCP meetings: November 12-16, 1997, Annual Meeting, Philadelphia, PA; May 16-20, 1998, Geriatrics '98 and Midyear Conference, Orlando, FL.

American Society of Health-System Pharmacists
7272 Wisconsin Avenue
Bethesda, MD 20814
(301) 657-3000

Helps patients make the best use of medications by offering a broad array of services and products to health-system pharmacists. Serves as a national accrediting organization for pharmacy residency and technician training programs. Publishes the *American Journal of Health-System Pharmacy, ASHP Newsletter*, and *International Pharmaceutical Abstracts*, among other publications.

Student memberships are open to individuals in undergraduate and graduate programs as well as recent graduates. Student chapters are located at many schools and colleges of pharmacy. Benefits include *Studentline*, a student newsletter; special programs at ASHP national meetings; and reduced meeting registration rates.

Upcoming ASHP meetings: December 7-11, 1997, Midyear Clinical Meeting, Atlanta, GA; May 31-June 4, 1998, Annual Meeting, Baltimore, MD.

National Community Pharmacists Association (formerly NARD)
205 Daingerfield Road
Alexandria, VA 22314
(703) 683-8200

Represents the professional and proprietary interests of independent community pharmacists. Publishes *America's Pharmacist, NCPA Newsletter.*

Student membership information available by telephone.

National Pharmaceutical Association
The Courtyards
107 Kilmayne Drive, Suite C
Cary, NC 27511
(800) 944-6742

Represents African-American pharmacists in all practice settings. Purpose is to plan and execute programs to improve the health, educational, and social environment of the community and to provide opportunities for professional development.

The Student National Pharmaceutical Association (SNPhA) has more than 500 members in 38 chapters at pharmacy schools nationwide. Benefits include a newsletter, updates on current pharmacy issues, scholarships and internships, and career placement assistance. SNPhA's telephone number is 904-561-2024.

Upcoming NPhA meetings: August 1-5, 1997, New Orleans, LA; July 24-28, 1998, Charleston, SC.

Organizations with Institutional Members

Generic Pharmaceutical Industry Association
1620 I Street, NW, Suite 800
Washington, DC 20006
(202) 833-9070

Open to manufacturers and distributors of generic drugs and industry supplies. Purpose is to increase recognition and use of generic pharmaceuticals.

National Association of Boards of Pharmacy
700 Busse Highway
Park Ridge, IL 60068
(847) 698-6227

Oversees licensure and relicensure of pharmacists in the United States. Publications include *NABP Newsletter* and *NAPLEX Candidates' Review Guide*.

Upcoming NABP meeting: May 16-20, 1998, 94th Annual Meeting, Orlando, FL. For more information about NABP, see Chapter 7.

National Association of Chain Drug Stores
413 North Lee Street
P.O. Box 1417-D49
Alexandria, VA 22313-1480
(703) 549-3001

Focuses on operational and professional interests of concern to the chain drug industry. Keeps Congress and federal agencies informed of issues affecting the industry. Members include retail chain community pharmacy companies; associate members include manufacturers, wholesalers, and companies that supply goods and services to chain community pharmacies. The NACDS Education Foundation awards scholarships and grants to support research and education. Periodicals include *NACDS Issues Update* and *NACDS Chain Pharmacist Practice Memo*.

National Association of Pharmaceutical Manufacturers
320 Old Country Road
Garden City, NY 11530

(516) 741-3699

Open to manufacturers of finished dosage forms (active member) and suppliers of bulk pharmaceuticals, goods, and services to the industry (associate member). Keeps members abreast of legislation affecting the industry; tracks regulatory issues; sponsors educational seminars and symposia.

Other Pharmaceutical Organizations

American Council on
Pharmaceutical Education
311 W. Superior Street,
Suite 512
Chicago, IL 60610
(312) 664-3575

An autonomous board that accredits pharmacy programs leading to the baccalaureate and doctor of pharmacy degrees and approves providers of continuing education.

National Council on Patient
Information and Education
666 11th Street, NW, Suite 110
Washington, DC 20001
(202) 347-6711

Coalition of consumer, health care, and pharmaceutical industry groups. Works to improve communication on medication therapy.

National Council of State
Pharmacy Association
Executives
P.O. Box 151
Chapel Hill, NC 27514-0151
(800) 852-3343

Members are executive officers of state pharmacy associations. Helps members improve management skills; surveys members on state pharmacy association activities.

United States Pharmacopeial
Convention, Inc.
12601 Twinbrook Parkway
Rockville, MD 20852
(301) 816-8299

Promotes the public health by establishing and disseminating standards for quality and authoritative information on the use of medications. Maintains databases; monitors reference standards; produces consumer drug references.

Offers summer internships to students in the health professions as well as a fellowship program. Call the Office of External Affairs at (301) 816-8282.

Internet Addresses of Pharmacy and Other Health Organizations

Here are the Internet addresses of several national pharmacy and health-related organizations. The associations are presented in alphabetical order.

All addresses begin with "http://".

American Academy of Family
Physicians: www.aafp.org

American Academy of
Pediatrics: www.aap.org

American Association of
Colleges of Pharmacy:
www.aacp.org

American Cancer Society:
www.cancer.org

American College of Clinical
Pharmacy: www.accp.com

American College of
Physicians: www.acponline.org

American Council on
Pharmaceutical Education:
76074.2703@compuserve.com

American Dental Association:
www.ada.org

American Diabetes Association:
www.diabetes.com

American Dietetic Association:
www.eatright.org

American Heart Association:
www.amhrt.org

American Institute of the
History of Pharmacy:
aihp@macc.wisc.edu

American Lung Association:
www.lungusa.org

American Medical Association:
www.ama-assn.org

American Nurses Association:
www.ana.org

American Pharmaceutical
Association: www.aphanet.org
American Psychological
Association: www.apa.org

American Society of
Consultant Pharmacists:
www.ascp.com

American Society of Health-
System Pharmacists:
www.ashp.com and
students@ashp.org

Institute for Safe Medication
Practices: www.ismp.org

National Association for Home
Care: www.nahc.org

National Council of State
Pharmacy Association
Executives:
Meba3@aol.com

National Pharmaceutical
Association:
bacm@interpath.com

United States Pharmacopeial
Convention, Inc.: www.usp.org

Appendix D

State Pharmacy Associations

David Laven, R.Ph.
Executive Director
Alabama Pharmacy Association
1211 Carmichael Way
Montgomery, AL 36106-3672
(334) 271-4222 FAX: (334) 271-5423

Erin Carey Byrne, R.Ph.
Executive Director
Alaska Pharmaceutical Association
Box 10-1185
Anchorage, AK 99510
(907) 563-8880 FAX: (907) 563-7880

Kathy Boyle
Executive Director
Arizona Pharmacy Association
1845 East Southern Avenue
Tempe, AZ 85282-5831
(602) 838-3385 FAX: (602) 838-3557

Richard E. Beck, R.Ph., CAE
Executive Vice President
Arkansas Pharmacists Association
417 South Victory
Little Rock, AR 72201
(501) 372-5250 FAX: (501) 372-0546

Chief Executive Officer
California Pharmacists Association
1112 "I" Street, Suite 200
Sacramento, CA 95814
(916) 444-7811 FAX: (916) 444-7929

Val Kalnins, R.Ph.
Executive Director
Colorado Pharmacists Association
5150 East Yale Circle
Suite 304
Denver, CO 80222
(303) 756-3069 FAX: (303) 756-3649

Marc S. McQuaid
Executive Vice President
Connecticut Pharmacists Association
35 Cold Spring Road, Suite 125
Rocky Hill, CT 06067
(860) 563-4619 FAX: (860) 257-8241

Martin Golden, R.Ph.
Executive Director
Delaware Pharmaceutical Society
1601 Milltown Road, Suite 8
Wilmington, DE 19711
(302) 892-2880 FAX: (302) 653-7800

James F. Harris, R.Ph.
Executive Director
DC Pharmaceutical Association
6406 Georgia Avenue, N.W., Suite 202
Washington, DC 20012
(202) 829-1515 FAX: (202) 829-1515

Michael Jackson, R.Ph.
Executive Vice President
Florida Pharmacy Association
610 North Adams Street
Tallahassee, FL 32301
(904) 222-2400 FAX: (904) 561-6758
Website: http:\\www.pharmview.com
E-Mail: mtg584@aol.com

Buddy Harden
Executive Vice President
Georgia Pharmacy Association
P.O. Box 95527
Atlanta, GA 30347
(404) 231-5074 FAX (404) 237-8435

Sue-Ann Yasuoka, R.Ph.
Executive Director
Hawaii Pharmaceutical Association
Box 1198
Honolulu, HI 96807
(808) 832-8810 FAX (808) 943-1738
E-Mail: yasuoka@gte.net

JoAn Condie
Executive Director
Idaho State Pharmacy Association
1365 North Orchard Street, Suite 316
Boise, ID 83706
(208) 376-2273 FAX (208) 376-5814

Executive Director
Illinois Pharmacists Association
223 West Jackson Boulevard, Suite 1000
Chicago, IL 60606
(312) 939-7300 FAX (312) 939-7220

Lawrence J. Sage
Executive Vice President
Indiana Pharmacists Association
729 North Pennsylvania Street
Indianapolis, IN 46204-1191
(317) 634-4968 FAX: (317) 632-1219

Thomas R. Temple, R.Ph., M.S.
Executive Vice President
Iowa Pharmacists Association
8515 Douglas Avenue, Suite 16
Des Moines, IA 50322
(515) 270-0713 FAX: (515) 270-2979
E-Mail: ipa@netins.net

Robert R. Williams, M.S., CAE
Executive Director
Kansas Pharmacists Association
1308 West 10th Street
Topeka, KS 66604
(913) 232-0439 FAX: (913) 232-3764

Robert L. Barnett Jr., R.Ph.
Executive Director
Kentucky Pharmacists Association
1228 U.S. Highway 127 South
Frankfort, KY 40601-4330
(502) 227-2303 FAX: (502) 227-2258

Christy Gabour Atwood
Executive Director
Louisiana Pharmacists Association
P.O. Box 14446
Baton Rouge, LA 70898-4446
(504) 926-2666 FAX: (504) 926-1020

Stanley Stewart, R.Ph.
Executive Director
Maine Pharmacy Association
P.O. Box 817
Bangor, ME 04402-0817
(207) 947-0885 FAX: (207) 947-1046

Tracy Baroni, R.Ph.
Executive Director
Maryland Pharmacists Association
650 West Lombard Street
Baltimore, MD 21201
(410) 727-0746 FAX: (410) 727-2253

Linda E. Barry, M.P.P.
Executive Director
Massachusetts Pharmacy Association
5 Lexington Street, Suite 5
Waltham, MA 02154
(617) 736-0101 FAX: (617) 736-0080
Website:

Appendix D (cont.)

http:\\www.channel1.com\users\mpha
E-Mail: mpha@user1.channell1.com

Larry D. Wagenknecht, R.Ph.
Chief Executive Officer
Michigan Pharmacists Association
815 North Washington Avenue
Lansing, MI 48906
(517) 484-1466 FAX: (517) 484-4893

William E. Bond, M.A., CAE
Executive Director
Minnesota Pharmacists Association
2550 University Avenue W, # 320N
St. Paul, MN 55114
(612) 644-3566 FAX: (612) 644-3965

Bo Dalton, R.Ph.
Executive Director
Mississippi Pharmacists Association
341 Edgewood Terrace Drive
Jackson, MS 39206-6273
(601) 981-0416 FAX: (601) 981-0451

George L. Oestreich, M.P.A., R.Ph.
Executive Director
Missouri Pharmacy Association
211 East Capitol Avenue
Jefferson City, MO 65101
(573) 636-7522 FAX: (573) 636-7485

Jim Smith & Kathy McGowan
Executive Directors
Montana State Pharmaceutical Association
34 West 6th, Suite 1C
Helena, MT 59601
(406) 449-3843 FAX: (406) 443-1592

Thomas R. Dolan, R.Ph.
Executive Director
Nebraska Pharmacists Association
6221 South 58th Street, Suite A
Lincoln, NE 68516
(402) 420-1500 FAX: (402) 420-1406
E-Mail: m&p@npharm.org

Karen Peska
Executive Director
Nevada Pharmacists Association
3660 Baker Lane
Reno, NV 89509
(702) 826-3981 FAX: (702) 825-0785

Elizabeth Gower, R.Ph.
Acting Executive Director
New Hampshire Pharmacists Association
Two Eagle Square, Suite 400
Concord, NH 03301-4956
(603) 229-0292 FAX: (603) 224-7769

Executive Officer
New Jersey Pharmacists Association
3 Marlen Drive, #B
Robbinsville, NJ 08691-1604
(609) 584-9063 FAX: (609) 586-8186
E-Mail: NJPHARM@aol.com

Dale Tinker
Executive Director
New Mexico Pharmaceutical Association
4800 Zuni, S.E.
Albuquerque, NM 87108
(505) 265-8720 FAX: (505) 255-8476

Craig M. Burridge, M.S.
Executive Director
Pharmacists Society of the State of New York
Pine West Plaza IV
Washington Avenue Extension
Albany, NY 12205
(518) 869-6595 FAX: (518) 464-0618

A. H. Mebane III, R.Ph.
Executive Director
North Carolina Pharmaceutical Association
P. O. Box 151
Chapel Hill, NC 27514
(919) 967-2237 FAX: (919) 968-9430

Galen Jordre
Executive Secretary
North Dakota Pharmaceutical Association
405 East Broadway
P.O. Box 5008
Bismarck, ND 58502-5008
(701) 258-4968 FAX: (701) 258-9312

Ernest Boyd, P.D., CAE
Executive Director
Ohio Pharmacists Association
6037 Frantz Road, Suite 106
Dublin, OH 43017
(614) 798-0037 FAX: (614) 798-0978
Website: www.ohiopharmacists.org
E-Mail: opa@ohiopharmacists.org

John D. Donner, P.D.
Executive Director
Oklahoma Pharmacists Association
Box 18731
Oklahoma City, OK 73154
(405) 528-3338 FAX: (405) 528-1417

A.J. "Burt" Kwitzky, R.Ph.
Executive Director
Oregon State Pharmacists Association
1460 State Street
Salem, OR 97301
(503) 585-4887 FAX: (503) 378-9067

Carmen A. DiCello, R.Ph.
Executive Director
Pennsylvania Pharmacists Association
508 North Third Street
Harrisburg, PA 17101-1199
(717) 234-6151 FAX: (717) 236-1618
Website: www.papharmacists.com
E-Mail: ppa@papharmacists.com

Felix Mendez
Executive Director
Colegio de Farmaceuticos de Puerto Rico
P.O. Box 360206

San Juan, PR 00936-0206
(809) 753-7167 FAX: (809) 759-9793

Donald Fowler
Executive Director
Rhode Island Pharmacists Association
Independence Square
500 Prospect Street
Pawtucket, RI 02860
(401) 725 4141 FAX: (401) 725-9960

James Bracewell
Executive Director
South Carolina Pharmacy Association
1405 Calhoun Street
Columbia, SC 29201
(803) 254-1065 FAX: (803) 254-9379
E-Mail: SCPhA@aol.com

Earl McKinstry
Acting Executive Director
South Dakota Pharmaceutical Association
Box 518
Pierre, SD 57501
(605) 224-2338 FAX: (605) 224-1280

Baeteena Black, D.Ph.
Executive Director
Tennessee Pharmacists Association
226 Capitol Boulevard, Suite 810
Nashville, TN 37219
(615) 256-3023 FAX: (615) 255-3528
E-Mail: TnPharm@aol.com

Paul F. Davis, R.Ph., CAE
Executive Director
Texas Pharmacy Association
P. O. Box 14709
Austin, TX 78761
(512) 836-8350 FAX: (512) 836-0308
E-Mail: TPA.PDAVIS@Juno.Com
Website: www.txpharmacy.com

Appendix D (cont.)

C. Neil Jensen, R.Ph.
Executive Director
Utah Pharmaceutical Association
1850 South Columbia Lane
Orem, UT 84058-8036
(801) 762-0452 FAX: (801) 762-0454

Fred H. Dobson III, R.Ph.
Executive Director
Vermont Pharmacists Association
P.O. Box 790
Richmond, VT 05477
(802) 434-3001 FAX: (802) 434-4803

Rebecca Snead, R.Ph.
Executive Director
Virginia Pharmacists Association
5501 Patterson Avenue, Suite 200
Richmond, VA 23226
(804) 285-4145 FAX: (804) 285-4227

Rod Shafer, R.Ph.
Executive Director
Washington State Pharmacists Association
1420 Maple Avenue, S.W., Suite 101
Renton, WA 98055-3196
(206) 228-7171 FAX: (206) 277-3897

Richard D. Stevens, J.D.
Executive Director
West Virginia Pharmacists Association
300 Capitol Street
Kanawha Valley Building, Suite 1002
Charleston, WV 25301
(304) 344-5302 FAX: (304) 344-5316

Chris Decker, R.Ph.
Executive Vice President
Wisconsin Pharmacists Association
701 Heartland Trail
Madison, WI 53717
(608) 827-9200 FAX: (608) 827-9292

Keith Sande, R.Ph.
Acting Executive Director
Wyoming Pharmacists Association
P.O. Box 541
Powell, WY 82435
(307) 754-4284

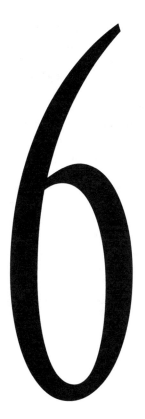

Chapter 6

Continuing Your Education: Residencies and Fellowships

Linda K. Ohri

Introduction

A bachelor of science or Pharm.D. degree prepares you for general pharmacy practice. If you want to specialize in a certain topic (e.g., pharmacokinetics or infectious disease) or practice arena (e.g., ambulatory care or home health care) or in the care of a specific patient population (e.g., children or the elderly), an experiential education program can enhance your skills, confidence, and marketability. These programs will also help prepare you for a career in academia or as a clinical educator and researcher.

Pharmacy offers two main types of postgraduate experiential program: residencies and fellowships. This chapter explores these two avenues of professional development.

Residency and Fellowship Programs

A pharmacy residency is an organized, directed, postgraduate training program in a defined area of pharmacy practice.[1-3] Residencies are offered in general pharmacy practice and in a number of different specialty practice areas. Residency programs emphasize the development of advanced practice skills. A residency may be undertaken at any point after receiving an entry-level degree in pharmacy.

Linda K. Ohri, Pharm.D., is Assistant Professor of Pharmacy Practice, Creighton University School of Pharmacy and Allied Health Professions, and Manager, Pediatric Drug Information Service, Children's Hospital, Omaha, Nebraska. For more information, she may be reached over the Internet (lohri@creighton.edu) or by phone (402-280-2951).

Most residency programs last one year; some, two years. Residents receive a stipend.

A pharmacy fellowship is an individualized postgraduate program that prepares the participant to become an independent researcher.[1-3] Fellowship programs emphasize the development of clinical research skills, although the fellow is also expected to continue to acquire advanced practice skills in his or her area of specialization. Fellowships are usually undertaken after a pharmacist has completed a residency or gained equivalent clinical experience. They are usually two years in length; some last only one year. These programs also provide a stipend.

Training Sites

Most residency and fellowship programs have a formal or informal affiliation with an academic health center; however, the primary training site is generally a practice institution (e.g., a hospital, ambulatory clinic, community pharmacy, home health care group, or other site).

Application Process

If you are interested in a specific residency or fellowship program, you must contact the designated program contact person for information. The names of these individuals appear in a variety of reference guides listed at the end of this chapter. You must submit your application directly to this individual. Most programs also require an onsite interview.

Accreditation of Residency and Fellowship Programs

Residencies

Approximately two thirds of all residency programs in the United States are accredited by the American Society of Health-System Pharmacists (ASHP). ASHP accredits a general pharmacy practice residency and 14 specialized residencies. There is no accreditation process currently in force for community pharmacy residencies; however, the American Pharmaceutical Association has recently released new guidelines for the design of such programs. The Canadian Society of Hospital Pharmacists (CaSHP) accredits most Canadian programs. The accreditation process requires that the institution sponsoring the residency document that it offers an organized, directed experiential curriculum. Accreditation reviews are conducted on site by a trained team of pharmacists who are experts in the focus area of the applicant program.

If a residency program is unaccredited, there may be several reasons. Some programs may simply be too new to be eligible for accreditation. Their focus may not fit within one of the 14 ASHP accreditation categories, or their administrators may choose not to seek accreditation. While an unaccredited residency may offer a high-quality educational experience, prospective applicants should examine such programs carefully to be sure that they will provide the desired learning opportunities. Comparing the written residency descriptions for the program of interest with general and specific standards set for accredited residencies in a similar focus area may be helpful.[1,4]

Table 1 lists the primary focus categories for all accredited residencies in the United States and Canada and for those nonaccredited residency or fellowship categories used by at least 10 programs.

Fellowships

There is no accreditation process for pharmacy fellowships in the United States or Canada. However, the American College of Clinical Pharmacy (ACCP) has published *ACCP*

Table 1

Pharmacy Residencies and Fellowships

Focus Categories
(Number of programs with the indicated primary focus or secondary emphasis)

- *Administration (46)
- *Ambulatory/Primary Care (101)
- Cardiology (41)
- Community Pharmacy (11)
- *Critical Care (68)
- *Drug Information (40)
- Drug Research (19)
- **General Hospital (54)
- *Geriatrics (28)
- *Infectious Disease (72)
- *Internal Medicine (39)
- Managed Care (23)
- Nephrology (13)
- Neurology (13)
- *Nuclear Pharmacy (4)
- *Nutrition (21)
- *Oncology (43)
- *Pediatrics (49)
- Pharmaceutical Care (28)
- Pharmacoeconomics (40)
- *Pharmacokinetics (74)
- Pharmacotherapy (17)
- *Pharmacy Practice (266)
- *Psychiatry (30)
- Transplantation (18)

* U.S. accredited residencies.
** Canadian accredited residencies.

Note: This table is a list of primary focus categories for all accredited residencies in the United States and Canada, and for those nonaccredited residency or fellowship categories used by at least 10 programs.

Guidelines for Research Fellowship Training Programs that fellowship preceptors are encouraged to follow.[2] A number of fellowship preceptors also submit their programs to a voluntary peer review process conducted by the ACCP Fellowship Review Committee. For more information about standards for fellowship programs, contact ACCP at (816) 531-2177.

ASHP Resident Matching Program

Most accredited general pharmacy practice residency programs in the United States participate in the ASHP Resident Matching Program. This program offers a formal process for "matching" residency applicants and programs. The applicant and the programs to which he or she has applied each submit a ranked-order list of those programs/applicants with which each is willing to match. The matching program then compares the lists of the program and applicant and "matches" the top choices of each.

The deadline for applying to participate in the Resident Matching Program is mid-January of each year. Applicants must submit their rank list by early March. They are informed of their status by the end of March.

For more information about this program, contact ASHP at (301) 657-3000.

Accredited specialized residency programs, nonaccredited residencies, and fellowships do not participate in the matching program.

Characteristics of Residency and Fellowship Programs

Appendixes E and F, located at the end of the chapter, list

the residencies and fellowships offered for the 1997-98 academic year. This information is drawn from RESFILE, a database that provides comprehensive information on residency and fellowship programs.[5,6]

The following information about residency and fellowship programs is based on a report describing U.S. and Canadian residencies and fellowships offered in 1995-6.[7] A total of 668 programs—540 residencies and 128 fellowships—were identified. All but 50 programs were in the United States. Seventy percent of the U.S. residencies were accredited. Of these, approximately two thirds were in pharmacy practice and one third were in specialized areas.

Positions Available

Most residencies begin in July and end in June of the following year. Fellowships typically last two years; they also begin in July and end in June. Pharmacy practice residency programs have an average of 2.4 positions each; most specialized residencies and fellowships offer one position annually.

Stipends and Benefits

The average stipend for U.S. residencies is about $25,000; the average fellowship stipend is around $24,000. Fellows may also receive some grant support. Geographic location is the strongest determinant of stipend level. A second factor is program focus; administrative residencies or fellowships tend to provide the highest stipends.

Most residency and fellowship programs offer health insurance, sick leave, and vacation benefits, as well as support for attending at least one national professional meeting annually.

Some residents and fellows may obtain deferments of college loan payments. These policies are determined by the applicant's lender. If this is a concern for you, ask questions about it as soon as you begin exploring your educational options or, better yet, when applying for your loan.

Elements of Residency and Fellowship Training

Residency programs focus on developing advanced practice skills in a general or specialized area of pharmaceutical care. Residents provide direct patient care in inpatient and ambulatory adult, pediatric, and geriatric units, as well as in specialty practice areas such as critical care, pharmacokinetics, and infectious disease. In pharmacy practice and some specialty programs, residents gain administrative and system management experience. They provide inservice education sessions, clerkship education, and patient education. Each resident also develops and carries out a research project during his or her training. Other areas of training are program specific.

For further information about the required elements of accredited U.S. residency programs, review *ASHP Opportunities '97*,[3] *Practice Standards of ASHP*,[4] and the *Residency Directory*.[1] These guidelines are also useful resources for individuals considering a nonaccredited residency.

Fellowship programs include many of the same elements as residency programs; however, they focus primarily on training in developing and carrying out a program of independent research. Activities include preparing and submitting grant proposals, developing a clinical research protocol, submitting the protocol to the institutional review committee, and carrying out the research project.

For more details on the fellowship experience, see the *ACCP Residency and Fellowship Directory*.[2]

Benefits of Residency and Fellowship Training

On successful completion of a residency or fellowship, you will be awarded a certificate by the institution offering the program. Most employers recognize these certificates as proof that the recipient has the advanced skills and knowledge needed to assume a position of leadership. More and more employers, such as those in academia, expect applicants to have residency and fellowship training.

Residency or fellowship graduates who have demonstrated leadership abilities are strong candidates for administrative positions in practice organizations. Such individuals may also be hired to develop and implement new patient care services. If you have your sights set on a position in clinical research, a fellowship will prepare you far better than entry-level, or even some other graduate level, programs. Individuals who wish to enter academia will benefit from the opportunity to participate in teaching pharmacy students during their training as well as the experience of providing interprofessional educational offerings.

It is important to be aware that some employers may not be prepared to pay the salaries that residency or fellowship graduates may command. If you are considering a residency or fellowship, you must assess the benefits of such training against the realities of employment opportunities in the area where you plan to practice. In general, however, the more training you have, the better. Over the course of an individual's career, there is evidence that postgraduate experiential education has a positive impact on the rate and level of professional advancement.[8-18]

Other benefits of residency and fellowship training have been discussed.[1,19] The benefit most mentioned by program graduates is the opportunity for a period of very intensive practice or research experience under the tutelage of a mentor. Former residents report that residency training increased their knowledge, skills, and confidence. It helped clarify their vision for where they wanted to proceed in the practice of their profession. They also note that they are more prepared to be a full member of the health care team. Graduates also speak highly of the leadership training gained and professional contacts made during training.[17,18]

Preparing for a Residency or Fellowship

When to Start

It is never too early (or too late!) to begin preparing for a residency or fellowship program. If you are just entering pharmacy training, find out as much as you can about different practice and other employment opportunities available to pharmacy graduates. As you identify areas of special interest, inquire about the educational requirements for these positions.

Consider developing a 5- and 10-year career plan. Good preparation will enhance your chances of being accepted by your program of choice. Appendix G is a time line that can help you plan.

Requirements and Qualifications

About half of the residencies are available to B.S. graduates; the others generally require a Pharm.D. or M.S. degree. Most fellowships require training beyond the entry-level degree as a prerequisite.

You will need to be diligent

in pursuit of academic excellence, but grades are not the only criterion by which residency or fellowship applicants are evaluated. Your performance in clerkships is of special interest to residency or fellowship program administrators. Letters of reference from clinical faculty who have supervised your clerkships are important. Successful completion of independent-study research demonstrates your interests and abilities, as do scholarly presentations and publications.

Don't forget leadership in professional organizations and association activities. These demonstrate motivation and abilities in service to the profession. Your pharmacy internship experience will give your prospective residency or fellowship program administrator, as well as you, an idea of how you respond to the demands of pharmacy practice. Other work, volunteer, and personal life experience can demonstrate many other desirable traits in a residency or fellowship applicant. Whether you decide to pursue experiential training, other educational endeavors, or employment, these activities will serve you well.

How to Learn about Residencies and Fellowships

Many schools of pharmacy offer formal and informal opportunities for students to learn about opportunities in postgraduate experiential education. Methods include lectures, counseling, and student forums.[20-22] If your school or college does not have such a forum, consider working with faculty members or student leaders to develop one.

Faculty advisers, residency and fellowship preceptors, and pharmacists practicing in your area of special interest are useful resources. Current residents and fellows, as well as those who have recently completed such programs, may also be helpful.

Many pharmacy associations offer residency forums or showcases in conjunction with their annual meetings. For example, the American Pharmaceutical Association Annual Meeting offers forums where students can learn about all types of postgraduate education programs, including residency and fellowship information. State associations may also offer such opportunities. Check with student or faculty representatives of these organizations on your campus about the times and sites for these programs.

The ASHP Midyear Clinical Meeting offers many opportunities to learn about residencies and fellowships. If you are seriously considering entering one of these programs, you should plan to attend. This meeting, held annually in early December, also provides an opportunity for prospective applicants and residency or fellowship representatives to meet prior to formal applications in January. *ASHP Opportunities '97* discusses the various programs offered at the Midyear Meeting.[3] The Midyear Clinical Meeting Program lists the times and places of specific events for those seeking residencies and fellowships.

Other resources are listed at the end of this chapter.

RESFILE: Simplifying the Search

RESFILE is a convenient, interactive source of thorough, up-to-date information on residencies and fellowships. It is a software package that provides information about accredited and nonaccredited programs in the United States and Canada.[5,6,23] All programs that the authors could identify have been entered into the RESFILE database. RESFILE was developed and is maintained at the Creighton University School of Pharmacy and Allied Health Professions, Omaha, Nebraska. Partial funding of the project has been provided by APhA and Merck.

The RESFILE software is distributed each September to the APhA-ASP faculty representative at each school or college of pharmacy. The software may be loaded on computers for student laboratories, faculty advisers, or students' own personal computers. There is no restriction on copying this software for student use. The RESFILE database may be loaded on any IBM-compatible personal computer with at least a 386 processor. It requires approximately 3.8 Mb of memory.

You may also download RESFILE software from the Internet (http://telemachus@creighton.edu or http://www.aphanet.org).

The program is user friendly. The software contains a help section, and print orientation materials are enclosed with the package. One school has trained students to provide brief training of other students who are interested in using this resource.[22]

RESFILE offers a number of convenient features to assist users in assessing their training options. Programs of potential interest may be identified on the basis of primary focus, location, accreditation status, residency or fellowship status, and availability to B.S. graduates. Appendix H shows a sample RESFILE program record.

Students may also use the software to generate letters of inquiry. The letters may be printed directly from the database or downloaded for revision in the student's computer. Appendix I provides an example of a RESFILE-generated inquiry letter.

Resources

Publications

• *ACCP Residency and Fellowship Directory*

Provides information about residencies and fellowships offered by members of ACCP. Includes both nonaccredited and accredited programs. Indexes programs on the basis of primary focus type and location. Distributed in October to ACCP members and to the dean of each school of pharmacy. Call ACCP at (816) 531-2177 for further information.

• *ASHP Opportunities '97*

Provides general information and many facts about pharmacy residency programs. Includes a checklist of steps necessary to participate in the ASHP Resident Matching Program. Each school or college of pharmacy ASHP Information Network for Students (INS) faculty representative receives copies of this resource for distribution to students.

• *Residency Directory*

Provides information about ASHP-accredited residencies. Indexes programs by primary focus and location. A copy is sent each October to the dean and INS faculty representative at all schools and colleges of pharmacy. A copy is provided to all individuals who apply to participate in the ASHP Resident Matching Program.

• *Practice Standards of ASHP*

Provides detailed standards and guidelines describing required components of ASHP-accredited residencies. Copies are generally available from faculty at your academic institution or a hospital employer.

Copies of the three ASHP references may also be purchased from ASHP at (301) 657-3000.

Computer Software

RESFILE 97. Obtain from APhA-ASP faculty adviser or download from the World Wide Web (http://telemachus@creighton.edu or http://www.aphanet.org).

References

1. *Residency Directory*. Bethesda, MD: American Society of Health-System Pharmacists; 1996.

2. *ACCP Residency and Fellowship Directory*. Kansas City, MO: American College of Clinical Pharmacy; 1996.

3. *ASHP Opportunities '97*. Bethesda, MD: American Society of Health-System Pharmacists; 1996.

4. *Practice Standards of ASHP*. Bethesda, MD: American Society of Health-System Pharmacists; 1996.

5. RESFILE '97. Software. Omaha, NE: Creighton University; 1996.

6. Cataldo R. Residencies database. *Am Pharm*. 1994;NS34(Aug):24-5.

7. Ohri LK, Pincus KT, Brantley HT. US and Canadian pharmacy residencies and fellowships: 1995. *Ann Pharmacotherapy*. 1995;28:1028-34.

8. Sauer BL, Koda-Kimble MA, Herfindal ET, et al. Evaluating curricular outcomes by use of a longitudinal alumni survey: Influence of gender and residency training. *Am J Pharm Educ*. 1994;58(1):16-24.

9. Herfindal ET, Koda-Kimble MA, Bernstein LR, et al. Effect of postgraduate training on the careers of University of California Pharm.D. graduates. *Am J Hosp Pharm*. 1987;44:536-43.

10. Knapp KK. Entry-level pharmacy positions in the 1990s: Taking manpower into consideration. *Pharm Bus*. Summer 1992;3:8-10.

11. Knapp KK, Letendre DE. Educational differentiation of the pharmacy workforce. *Am J Hosp Pharm*. 1989;46:2476-82.

12. Knapp KK, Sorby DL. The impact of specialization on pharmacy manpower. *Am J Hosp Pharm*. 1991;47:2665-95.

13. Koda-Kimble MA, Herfindal ET, Shimomura SK, et al. Practice patterns, attitudes, and activities of University of California Pharm.D. graduates. *Am J Hosp Pharm*. 1985;42:2463-71.

14. Lopez J. Pharmacy residencies: A preceptor's perspective. *Cal J Hosp Pharm*. 1989;1:8-9.

15. Ray MD. Pharmacy manpower revisited (part I). *Cal J Hosp Pharm*. 1993;5(March):5-9.

16. Vogel D, Blake A. Why pursue a residency? *Am J Hosp Pharm*. 1991;48:1878.

17. Pierpaoli PG. Mentoring. *Am J Hosp Pharm*. 1992;49:2175-8.

18. Pierpaoli PG. Mentors and residency training. *Am J Hosp Pharm*. 1990;47:116-7.

19. Bucci KK, Knapp KK, Ohri LK, et al. Factors motivating pharmacy students to pursue residency and fellowship training. *Am J Health-Syst Pharm*. 1995;52:2696-701.

20. Lum BL, Cox D. Helping clerkship students apply for residencies. *Am J Health-Syst Pharm*. 1995;52:209-10.

21. Bucci KK, Teat DW. Promoting postgraduate programs in a residency forum. *Am J Hosp Pharm*. 1992;49:1396.

22. Knapp KK. Promoting residencies to pharmacy students. *Am J Hosp Pharm*. 1991;48:1717-21.

23. Ohri LK, Pincus KT. Computerized database for residency and fellowship programs. *Am J Hosp Pharm*. 1993;50:1137-8.

Appendix E

RESFILE 97 Residencies

State or Province	Primary Focus	Site	Accred. Status	In ASHP Matching Program?	City	Contact Phone	RESFILE Record #
USA							
Alabama	DRUG INFORMATION	Univ of Alabama Hosp	ASHP	N	Birmingham	(205) 934-2162	529
	DRUG INFORMATION	Samford Univ	NO	N	Birmingham	(205) 870-2891	1065
	INTERNAL MEDICINE	Birmingham Baptist Med Ctr, Princeton	ASHP	N	Birmingham	(205) 783-3474	1348
	MANAGED CARE	Samford Univ, Managed Care Institute	NO	N	Birmingham	(205) 870-2988	1066
	NUTRITION	Huntsville Hosp	NO	N	Huntsville	(205) 517-8288	1162
	PHARMACY PRACTICE	Univ of Alabama Hosp	ASHP	Y	Birmingham	(205) 934-4628	151
	PHARMACY PRACTICE	Huntsville Hosp	ASHP	Y	Huntsville	(205) 517-8288	858
Arkansas	AMBULATORY/PRIMARY CARE	VA Med Ctr-Little Rock	NO	N	Little Rock	(501) 671-2531	1226
	MANAGED CARE	Pharmacy Associates, Inc	NO	N	Little Rock	(501) 221-2330	1446
	PHARMACY PRACTICE	Arkansas Children's Hosp	ASHP	Y	Little Rock	(501) 320-1449	824
	PHARMACY PRACTICE	The Univ Hosp of Arkansas	ASHP	Y	Little Rock	(501) 686-6220	862
	PHARMACY PRACTICE	VA Med Ctr-Little Rock	ASHP	Y	Little Rock	(501) 660-2011	823
Arizona	AMBULATORY/PRIMARY CARE	USPHS Indian Hosp	ASHP	N	Whiteriver	(602) 338-4911	493
	COMMUNITY PHARMACY	Winslow Indian Health Clinic	NO	N	Winslow	(520) 289-4646	494
	CRITICAL CARE	Univ Med Ctr	NO	N	Tucson	(520) 694-5600	1433
	DRUG INFORMATION	Univ Med Ctr	ASHP	N	Tucson	(520) 694-2281	3
	NUTRITION	Univ Med Ctr	ASHP	N	Tucson	(602) 694-6127	958
	PHARMACY PRACTICE	Carl T Hayden VA Med Ctr	ASHP	Y	Phoenix	(602) 277-5551	384
	PHARMACY PRACTICE	Talbert Medical Management Corp/FHP Health Care	ASHP	Y	Phoenix	(602) 833-6041	1318
	PHARMACY PRACTICE	VA Med Ctr-Tucson	ASHP	Y	Tucson	(602) 629-1829	866
	PHARMACY PRACTICE	Tucson Med Ctr	ASHP	Y	Tucson	(602) 324-1882	999
	PHARMACY PRACTICE	Univ Med Ctr	ASHP	Y	Tucson	(520) 626-5349	865
	PSYCHIATRY	Univ of Arizona	NO	N	Tucson	(602) 626-5404	757
California	ADMINISTRATION	Kaiser Foundation Hosp	ASHP	N	Los Angeles	(213) 667-8306	876
	ADMINISTRATION	Cedars-Sinai Med Ctr	NO	N	Los Angeles	(310) 855-5611	1006
	ADMINISTRATION	The Med Ctr at UCSF	ASHP	N	San Francisco	(415) 476-5587	394
	ADMINISTRATION	Stanford Univ Hosp	ASHP	N	Stanford	(415) 723-5970	1002
	AMBULATORY/PRIMARY CARE	Kaiser Permanente	ASHP	N	Harbor City	(310) 517-2268	761
	AMBULATORY/PRIMARY CARE	Friendly Hills Healthcare Network	ASHP	N	La Habra	(310) 905-3072	1345
	AMBULATORY/PRIMARY CARE	Dept of VA Outpatient Clinic, LA	ASHP	N	Los Angeles	(213) 253-5119	398
	AMBULATORY/PRIMARY CARE	Univ of Southern California SOP	ASHP	N	Los Angeles	(213) 342-2648	397
	AMBULATORY/PRIMARY CARE	Cedars-Sinai Med Ctr	NO	N	Los Angeles	(310) 855-5611	1158
	AMBULATORY/PRIMARY CARE	VA Northern California System of Clinics	ASHP	N	Martinez	(510) 372-2380	259
	AMBULATORY/PRIMARY CARE	Univ of California, Davis Med Ctr	NO	N	Sacramento	(916) 734-0441	803

Appendix E (cont.)

State or Province	Primary Focus	Site	Accred. Status	In ASHP Matching Program?	City	Contact Phone	RESFILE Record #
	AMBULATORY/PRIMARY CARE	VA Med Ctr-San Diego	ASHP	N	San Diego	(619) 552-8585	1285
	AMBULATORY/PRIMARY CARE	Dept of VA Med Ctr-San Francisco	ASHP	N	San Francisco	(415) 750-2053	1222
	AMBULATORY/PRIMARY CARE	VA Med Ctr-Sepulveda	ASHP	N	Sepulveda	(818) 895-9341	1346
	DRUG INFORMATION	Kaiser Permanente Med Care Program/DIS	ASHP	N	Downey	(310) 803-2937	530
	DRUG INFORMATION	Univ of California, Irvine Med Ctr	ASHP	N	Orange	(714) 456-5514	965
	DRUG INFORMATION	Univ of California, San Francisco	ASHP	N	San Francisco	(415) 476-1733	160
	DRUG INFORMATION	Univ of the Pacific	NO	N	Stockton	(209) 946-2412	1437
	FAMILY PRACTICE	The Med Ctr at UCSF	NO	N	San Francisco	(415) 476-1972	961
	GERIATRICS	VA Med Ctr-West Los Angeles	ASHP	N	Los Angeles	(310) 268-3152	257
	GERIATRICS	VA Med Ctr-Sepulveda	ASHP	N	Sepulveda	(818) 895-9341	408
	HOME HEALTH CARE	The Med Ctr at UCSF	NO	N	San Francisco	(415) 476-3513	960
	INFECTIOUS DISEASE	Univ of California, San Francisco	NO	N	San Francisco	(415) 476-0892	963
	INTERNAL MEDICINE	Kern Med Ctr	ASHP	N	Bakersfield	(805) 326-2200	688
	ONCOLOGY	The Med Ctr at UCSF	ASHP	N	San Francisco	(415) 476-1230	962
	PEDIATRICS	Children's Hosp Los Angeles	NO	N	Los Angeles	(213) 669-2406	1352
	PEDIATRICS	Univ of Southern California SOP	ASHP	N	Los Angeles	(213) 342-2648	414
	PEDIATRICS	Univ of California, Davis Med Ctr	NO	N	Sacramento	(916) 734-3305	802
	PEDIATRICS	The Med Ctr at UCSF	ASHP	N	San Francisco	(415) 476-8364	415
	PHARMACOKINETICS	Univ of California, San Francisco	ASHP	N	San Francisco	(415) 476-8891	816
	PHARMACY PRACTICE	Kaiser Foundation Hosp, Anaheim	ASHP	Y	Anaheim	(714) 978-4706	869
	PHARMACY PRACTICE	Kaiser Permanente Med Ctr	ASHP	Y	Bellflower	(310) 461-6070	1319
	PHARMACY PRACTICE	City of Hope National Med Ctr	ASHP	Y	Duarte	(818) 301-8305	363
	PHARMACY PRACTICE	Kaiser Foundation Hosp, Fontana	ASHP	Y	Fontana	(909) 427-3838	362
	PHARMACY PRACTICE	Marin General Hosp	ASHP	Y	Greenbrae	(415) 925-7867	615
	PHARMACY PRACTICE	VA Med Ctr-Long Beach	ASHP	Y	Long Beach	(310) 494-5502	386
	PHARMACY PRACTICE	Long Beach Memorial Med Ctr	ASHP	Y	Long Beach	(310) 933-0250	79
	PHARMACY PRACTICE	Cedars-Sinai Med Ctr	ASHP	Y	Los Angeles	(310) 855-5611	364
	PHARMACY PRACTICE	Kaiser Foundation Hosp, Los Angeles	ASHP	Y	Los Angeles	(213) 667-8306	365
	PHARMACY PRACTICE	LAC + USC Med Ctr	ASHP	Y	Los Angeles	(213) 342-2648	387
	PHARMACY PRACTICE	USC Norris Cancer Ctr and Hosp	ASHP	Y	Los Angeles	(213) 764-3600	871
	PHARMACY PRACTICE	VA Med Ctr-West Los Angeles	ASHP	Y	Los Angeles	(310) 268-3150	407
	PHARMACY PRACTICE	Hosp of the Good Samaritan	ASHP	Y	Los Angeles	(213) 977-2313	720
	PHARMACY PRACTICE	Kaiser Permanente Med Ctr, West LA	ASHP	Y	Los Angeles	(213) 857-2157	872
	PHARMACY PRACTICE	UCLA Med Ctr	ASHP	Y	Los Angeles	(310) 206-6555	154
	PHARMACY PRACTICE	Hoag Memorial Hosp Presbyterian	ASHP	Y	Newport Beach	(714) 760-2098	41
	PHARMACY PRACTICE	St Joseph Hosp	ASHP	Y	Orange	(714) 771-8067	366
	PHARMACY PRACTICE	Univ of California, Irvine Med Ctr	ASHP	Y	Orange	(714) 456-5514	156
	PHARMACY PRACTICE	Desert Hosp, Palm Springs	ASHP	Y	Palm Springs	(619) 323-6228	991
	PHARMACY PRACTICE	Lucile Salter Packard Children's Hosp	ASHP	Y	Palo Alto	(415) 497-8781	989
	PHARMACY PRACTICE	VA Med Ctr-Palo Alto	ASHP	Y	Palo Alto	(415) 858-3968	260
	PHARMACY PRACTICE	Kaiser Foundation Hosp	ASHP	Y	Panorama City	(818) 375-2885	990
	PHARMACY PRACTICE	Huntington Memorial Hosp	ASHP	Y	Pasadena	(818) 397-5237	992
	PHARMACY PRACTICE	Univ of California, Davis Med Ctr	ASHP	Y	Sacramento	(916) 734-3305	371
	PHARMACY PRACTICE	San Bernardino County Med Ctr	ASHP	Y	San Bernardino	(909) 387-8140	367

Appendix E (cont.)

State or Province	Primary Focus	Site	Accred. Status	In ASHP Matching Program?	City	Contact Phone	RESFILE Record #
	PHARMACY PRACTICE	Naval Med Ctr	ASHP	N	San Diego	(619) 532-8401	368
	PHARMACY PRACTICE	VA Med Ctr-San Diego	ASHP	Y	San Diego	(619) 552-8585	466
	PHARMACY PRACTICE	Kaiser Foundation Hosp	ASHP	Y	San Diego	(619) 528-5383	710
	PHARMACY PRACTICE	Univ of California, San Diego Med Ctr	ASHP	Y	San Diego	(619) 543-6190	158
	PHARMACY PRACTICE	California Pacific Med Ctr	ASHP	Y	San Francisco	(415) 923-3206	120
	PHARMACY PRACTICE	Univ of California, San Francisco	ASHP	Y	San Francisco	(415) 476-5587	159
	PHARMACY PRACTICE	VA Med Ctr-San Francisco	ASHP	Y	San Francisco	(415) 221-4810	262
	PHARMACY PRACTICE	Stanford Univ Hosp	ASHP	Y	Stanford	(415) 723-5970	1001
	PHARMACY PRACTICE	St Joseph's Med Ctr of Stockton	ASHP	Y	Stockton	(209) 467-6518	613
	PHARMACY PRACTICE	David Grant US Air Force Med Ctr	ASHP	Y	Travis AFB	(707) 423-7132	988
	PHARMACY PRACTICE	Presbyterian Intercommunity Hosp	ASHP	Y	Whittier	(213) 698-0811	388
	PHARMACY PRACTICE	Kaiser Foundation Hosp	ASHP	Y	Woodland Hills	(818) 719-2910	1196
	PSYCHIATRY	Univ of Southern California SOP	ASHP	N	Los Angeles	(213) 342-2648	699
	TRANSPLANTATION	UCLA Med Ctr	NO	N	Los Angeles	(310) 206-4952	1302
Colorado	ADMINISTRATION	The Children's Hosp	NO	N	Denver	(303) 861-6834	835
	AMBULATORY/PRIMARY CARE	Kaiser Permanente	NO	N	Aurora	(303) 739-3545	1224
	AMBULATORY/PRIMARY CARE	VA Med Center	NO	N	Denver	(303) 393-2806	1425
	CRITICAL CARE	Univ Hospital	NO	N	Denver	(303) 270-5136	1434
	DRUG INFORMATION	Univ of Colorado Health Sciences Ctr	NO	N	Denver	(303) 270-8480	901
	NUTRITION	Univ of Colorado Health Sciences Ctr	NO	N	Denver	(303) 270-4547	308
	ONCOLOGY	Univ Hospital	NO	N	Denver	(303) 315-7709	1455
	PEDIATRICS	The Children's Hosp	ASHP	N	Denver	(303) 861-6834	719
	PHARMACY PRACTICE	Univ Hosp	ASHP	Y	Denver	(303) 270-7555	309
	PHARMACY PRACTICE	VA Med Ctr-Denver	ASHP	Y	Denver	(303) 393-2806	385
Connecticut	PEDIATRICS	Hartford Hosp	NO	N	Hartford	(203) 545-2003	1354
	PHARMACY PRACTICE	Univ of Connecticut Health Ctr/John Dempsey Hosp	ASHP	Y	Farmington	(203) 679-2988	297
	PHARMACY PRACTICE	Hartford Hosp	ASHP	Y	Hartford	(203) 545-2912	37
District of Columbia	ASSOCIATION MANAGEMENT	American Pharmaceutical Association	NO	N	Washington	(202) 429-7353	478
	NUCLEAR PHARMACY	Walter Reed Army Med Ctr	ASHP	N	Washington	(202) 782-5296	1222
	ONCOLOGY	Walter Reed Army Med Ctr	ASHP	N	Washington	(202) 782-0763	485
	PHARMACY PRACTICE	Children's National Med Ctr	NO	N	Washington	(202) 884-2055	18
	PHARMACY PRACTICE	Washington Hosp Ctr	ASHP	Y	Washington	(202) 877-7920	1320
	PHARMACY PRACTICE	Walter Reed Army Med Ctr	ASHP	N	Washington	(202) 782-0385	337
Florida	ADMINISTRATION	Shands Hosp	NO	N	Gainesville	(904) 395-0404	136
	AMBULATORY/PRIMARY CARE	Univ Med Ctr	ASHP	N	Jacksonville	(904) 549-4157	796
	AMBULATORY/PRIMARY CARE	Florida Hosp Family Practice Residency	ASHP	N	Orlando	(407) 897-5725	952
	AMBULATORY/PRIMARY CARE	James A Haley Veterans Hosp	ASHP	N	Tampa	(813) 972-2000	621
	CARDIOLOGY	Tampa General Hosp	NO	N	Tampa	(813) 251-7301	1357
	CRITICAL CARE	Shands Hosp Univ of Florida	ASHP	N	Gainesville	(352) 395-0404	817
	CRITICAL CARE	Univ Med Ctr	ASHP	N	Jacksonville	(904) 49-4157	1160
	CRITICAL CARE	Tampa General Hosp	NO	N	Tampa	(813) 251-7301	809
	DRUG INFORMATION	Shands Hosp Univ of Florida	ASHP	N	Gainesville	(352) 395-0408	654

Appendix E (cont.)

State or Province	Primary Focus	Site	Accred. Status	In ASHP Matching Program?	City	Contact Phone	RESFILE Record #
	DRUG INFORMATION	Univ Med Ctr	ASHP	N	Jacksonville	(904) 549-4157	797
	DRUG INFORMATION	Nova-Southeastern Univ	NO	N	North Miami Beach	(305) 949-4000	1355
	FAMILY PRACTICE	Univ of Florida Family Medicine	NO	N	Gainesville	(904) 392-4541	547
	GERIATRICS	VA Med Ctr-Gainesville	ASHP	N	Gainesville	(352) 374-6062	403
	INFECTIOUS DISEASE	VA Med Ctr-Miami	NO	N	Miami	(305) 324-3102	1242
	INTERNAL MEDICINE	VA Med Ctr-Gainesville	ASHP	N	Gainesville	(904) 374-6062	317
	INTERNAL MEDICINE	Shands Hosp	NO	N	Gainesville	(352) 395-0404	1443
	INTERNAL MEDICINE	Tampa General Hosp	NO	N	Tampa	(813) 251-7301	808
	NEUROLOGY	VA Hosp, Tacachale Community of Excellence, Tallahasse Mem.	NO	N	Gainesville	(352) 955-5926	1477
	NUTRITION	VA Med Ctr	NO	N	Gainesville	(904) 376-1611	1453
	ONCOLOGY	Shands Hosp	ASHP	N	Gainesville	(904) 395-0404	653
	ONCOLOGY	H Lee Moffitt Cancer Ctr and Research Institute	ASHP	N	Tampa	(813) 972-4673	995
	PAIN MANAGEMENT	Univ of South Florida	NO	N	Tampa	(813) 972-8456	1460
	PEDIATRICS	Shands Hosp	ASHP	N	Gainesville	(904) 395-0404	655
	PEDIATRICS	Miami Children's Hosp	ASHP	N	Miami	(305) 666-6511	313
	PEDIATRICS	All Children's Hosp	ASHP	N	St Petersburg	(813) 892-4365	411
	PHARMACY PRACTICE	Bay Pines VA Med Ctr	ASHP	Y	Bay Pines	(813) 398-9431	1197
	PHARMACY PRACTICE	Shands Hosp/Univ of Florida	ASHP	Y	Gainesville	(904) 395-0404	135
	PHARMACY PRACTICE	Univ Med Ctr	ASHP	Y	Jacksonville	(904) 549-4157	172
	PHARMACY PRACTICE	VA Med Ctr-Miami	ASHP	Y	Miami	(305) 324-3102	851
	PHARMACY PRACTICE	James A Haley Veterans' Hosp	ASHP	Y	Tampa	(813) 972-2000	264
	POISON CONTROL/TOXICOLOGY	Univ Med Ctr, Florida	NO	N	Jacksonville	(904) 549-4465	795
	PSYCHIATRY	Nova-Southeastern Univ	NO	N	Miami Beach	(305) 949-4000	1356
	TRANSPLANTATION	Shands Hosp	NO	N	Gainesville	(352) 395-0404	1473
Georgia	DRUG INFORMATION	Mercer Univ SOP	ASHP	N	Atlanta	(770) 986-3204	691
	NUTRITION	Emory Univ System of Healthcare	ASHP	N	Atlanta	(404) 712-7800	682
	ONCOLOGY	Emory Univ System of Healthcare	ASHP	N	Atlanta	(404) 712-4640	28
	PHARMACY PRACTICE	Piedmont Hosp/Mercer Univ	ASHP	Y	Atlanta	(404) 605-4205	553
	PHARMACY PRACTICE	Egleston Children's Hosp	ASHP	Y	Atlanta	(404) 325-6502	996
	PHARMACY PRACTICE	Emory Univ Hosp	ASHP	Y	Atlanta	(404) 712-4640	26
	PHARMACY PRACTICE	Med College of Georgia Hosp and Clinics	ASHP	Y	Augusta	(706) 721-3221	377
	PHARMACY PRACTICE	The Med Ctr Inc	ASHP	Y	Columbus	(706) 571-1495	930
	PHARMACY PRACTICE	Dekalb Med Ctr	ASHP	Y	Decatur	(404) 501-5152	318
	PHARMACY PRACTICE	Med Ctr of Central Georgia	ASHP	Y	Macon	(912) 633-1440	1404
	POISON CONTROL/TOXICOLOGY	Georgia Poison Ctr	NO	N	Atlanta	(404) 616-9237	1359
	PSYCHIATRY	Mercer Univ	ASHP	N	Atlanta	(404) 986-3211	689
Hawaii	PHARMACY PRACTICE	The Queen's Med Ctr	ASHP	Y	Honolulu	(808) 547-4736	122
	PHARMACY PRACTICE	Tripler Army Med Ctr	ASHP	N	Tripler AMC	(808) 433-5240	993
Idaho	AMBULATORY/PRIMARY CARE	VA Med Ctr-Boise	ASHP	N	Boise	(208) 389-7946	1307
	AMBULATORY/PRIMARY CARE	Idaho State Univ	NO	N	Pocatello	(208) 239-2682	1362
	FAMILY PRACTICE	Idaho State Univ	NO	N	Pocatello	(208) 236-3836	1363
	GERIATRICS	VA Med Ctr-Boise	ASHP	N	Boise	(208) 389-7946	47

Appendix E (cont.)

State or Province	Primary Focus	Site	Accred. Status	In ASHP Matching Program?	City	Contact Phone	RESFILE Record #
Illinois	ADMINISTRATION	Rush-Presbyterian-St Luke's Med Ctr	NO	N	Chicago	(312) 942-5989	391
	ADMINISTRATION	Univ of Illinois Hosp/Michael Reese Hosp	NO	N	Chicago	(312) 996-6300	174
	AMBULATORY/PRIMARY CARE	Univ of Illinois COP	ASHP	N	Chicago	(312) 996-6300	179
	AMBULATORY/PRIMARY CARE	Midwestern Univ	NO	N	Downers Grove	(630) 971-6417	1420
	DRUG INFORMATION	Univ of Illinois Hosp/Michael Reese Hosp	ASHP	N	Chicago	(312) 996-6300	176
	DRUG INFORMATION	Rush-Presbyterian-St Luke's Med Ctr	ASHP	N	Chicago	(312) 942-3210	642
	EMERGENCY MEDICINE	Univ of Illinois Hosp	NO	N	Chicago	(312) 996-5328	902
	INTERNAL MEDICINE	Rush-Presbyterian-St Luke's Med Ctr	ASHP	N	Chicago	(312) 942-6153	911
	NEPHROLOGY	University of IL at Chicago	NO	N	Chicago	(312) 996-0894	1450
	ONCOLOGY	Univ of IL at Chicago	NO	N	Chicago	(312) 996-0379	1456
	ONCOLOGY	Univ of Illinois Hosp/Michael Reese Hosp	NO	N	Chicago	(312) 996-0894	177
	PEDIATRICS	Univ of Illinois Hosp/Michael Reese Hosp	ASHP	N	Chicago	(312) 996-0895	178
	PHARMACOKINETICS	Univ of Illinois	NO	N	Chicago	(312) 413-8282	1367
	PHARMACOKINETICS	Univ of Illinois Hosp/Michael Reese Hosp	NO	N	Chicago	(312) 996-3341	184
	PHARMACY PRACTICE	St Elizabeth's Hosp/St Louis COP	ASHP	Y	Belleville	(800) 995-2120	826
	PHARMACY PRACTICE	West Side VA Med Ctr	ASHP	Y	Chicago	(312) 666-6500	379
	PHARMACY PRACTICE	Northwestern Memorial Hosp	ASHP	Y	Chicago	(312) 908-2546	103
	PHARMACY PRACTICE	VA Lakeside Med Ctr	ASHP	Y	Chicago	(312) 943-6600	1198
	PHARMACY PRACTICE	Univ of Illinois Hosp/Michael Reese Hosp	ASHP	Y	Chicago	(312) 996-0875	173
	PHARMACY PRACTICE	Rush-Presbyterian-St Luke's Med Ctr	ASHP	Y	Chicago	(312) 942-6153	378
	PHARMACY PRACTICE	Evanston Hosp Corp	ASHP	Y	Evanston	(847) 570-2203	1405
	PHARMACY PRACTICE	Lutheran General Hosp	ASHP	Y	Park Ridge	(847) 723-5398	55
	PHARMACY PRACTICE	St John's Hosp	ASHP	Y	Springfield	(217) 544-6464	143
	PSYCHIATRY	Univ of Illinois Hosp and Clinics	NO	N	Chicago	(312) 996-6300	668
	TRANSPLANTATION	Univ of Illinois	NO	N	Chicago	(312) 996-6300	1368
Indiana	DRUG INFORMATION	Purdue Univ SOP and Pharmacal Sciences	ASHP	N	West Lafayette	(317) 630-6896	1414
	INTERNAL MEDICINE	Purdue Univ and Indiana Univ Med Ctr	ASHP	N	Indianapolis	(317) 274-1895	482
	PEDIATRICS	James Whitcomb Riley Hosp for Children	NO	N	Indianapolis	(317) 274-5000	321
	PHARMACY PRACTICE	St Margaret Mercy North Campus	ASHP	Y	Hammond	(219) 933-2300	1321
	PHARMACY PRACTICE	St Vincent Hosp and Health Care Ctr	ASHP	Y	Indianapolis	(317) 338-2260	611
	PHARMACY PRACTICE	Indiana Univ Med Ctr	ASHP	Y	Indianapolis	(317) 274-1895	48
	PHARMACY PRACTICE	Methodist Hosp/Butler Univ	ASHP	Y	Indianapolis	(317) 929-3484	1322
Iowa	AMBULATORY/PRIMARY CARE	Iowa City VA Med Ctr	ASHP	N	Iowa City	(319) 339-7119	1183
	INFECTIOUS DISEASE	Univ of Iowa Hospitals and Clinics	NO	N	Iowa City	(319) 356-2577	1238
	ONCOLOGY	Univ of Iowa Clinical Cancer Ctr	NO	N	Iowa City	(319) 356-2577	1256
	PHARMACY PRACTICE	Univ of Iowa Hosp and Clinics	ASHP	Y	Iowa City	(319) 356-2577	189
Kansas	COMMUNITY PHARMACY	Univ of Kansas SOP	NO	N	Lawrence	(913) 864-4881	294
	DRUG INFORMATION	Univ of Kansas Med Ctr	ASHP	N	Kansas City	(913) 588-2303	983
	PHARMACY PRACTICE	Univ of Kansas Med Ctr	ASHP	Y	Kansas City	(913) 588-2330	191
Kentucky	CRITICAL CARE	Univ of Kentucky Med Ctr	ASHP	N	Lexington	(606) 323-6029	879
	ONCOLOGY	Univ of Kentucky Med Ctr	ASHP	N	Lexington	(606) 323-6029	883
	PEDIATRICS	Univ of Kentucky Med Ctr	ASHP	N	Lexington	(606) 323-6029	1161

Appendix E (cont.)

State or Province	Primary Focus	Site	Accred. Status	In ASHP Matching Program?	City	Contact Phone	RESFILE Record #
	PHARMACY PRACTICE	VA Med Ctr	ASHP	Y	Lexington	(606) 233-4511	1323
	PHARMACY PRACTICE	Univ of Kentucky Med Ctr	ASHP	Y	Lexington	(606) 323-6029	636
	PHARMACY PRACTICE	St Claire Med Ctr	ASHP	Y	Morehead	(606) 783-6740	192
	PSYCHIATRY	Eastern State Psychiatric Hosp	NO	N	Lexington	(606) 246-7537	1370
Louisiana	PHARMACY PRACTICE	VA Med Ctr-New Orleans	NO	N	New Orleans	(504) 589-5299	1324
	PHARMACY PRACTICE	Overton Brooks VA Med Ctr	ASHP	Y	Shreveport	(318) 424-6001	1325
Maryland	AMBULATORY/PRIMARY CARE	Univ of Maryland	NO	N	Baltimore	(410) 706-7338	1374
	AMBULATORY/PRIMARY CARE	Warren G Magnuson Clinic Ctr/NIH	ASHP	N	Bethesda	(301) 496-4363	979
	ASSOCIATION MANAGEMENT	American Society of Health-System Pharmacists	NO	N	Bethesda	(301) 657-3000	973
	CARDIOLOGY	Univ of Maryland	NO	N	Baltimore	(410) 706-7338	1375
	COMMUNITY PHARMACY	Univ of Maryland	NO	N	Baltimore	(410) 706-1865	1373
	CRITICAL CARE	Univ of Maryland Med System	ASHP	N	Baltimore	(410) 328-3720	489
	DRUG INFORMATION	Univ of Maryland	NO	N	Baltimore	(410) 706-7338	1376
	DRUG INFORMATION	WG Magnuson Clin Ctr/NIH	ASHP	N	Bethesda	(301) 496-4363	822
	INFECTIOUS DISEASE	Univ of Maryland	NO	N	Baltimore	(410) 706-7338	1377
	INTERNAL MEDICINE	Memorial Hospital at Easton	NO	N	Easton	(410) 822-1000	1441
	MANAGED CARE	Advance Paradigm Clinical Services Inc	NO	N	Hunt Valley	(410) 785-2182	1372
	NUTRITION	Univ of Maryland Med System	NO	N	Baltimore	(410) 328-5650	563
	ONCOLOGY	Univ of Maryland Cancer Ctr	NO	N	Baltimore	(410) 328-2563	1381
	ONCOLOGY	Warren G Magnuson Clinical Ctr/NIH	ASHP	N	Bethesda	(301) 496-4363	669
	PEDIATRICS	Johns Hopkins Hosp	ASHP	N	Baltimore	(410) 614-2949	920
	PHARMACOTHERAPY	Univ of Maryland	NO	N	Baltimore	(410) 706-7338	1379
	PHARMACY PRACTICE	Johns Hopkins Hosp	ASHP	Y	Baltimore	(410) 955-6591	51
	PHARMACY PRACTICE	Univ of Maryland Med System	ASHP	Y	Baltimore	(410) 328-5650	195
	PHARMACY PRACTICE	Warren G Magnuson Clin Ctr, NIH	ASHP	Y	Bethesda	(301) 496-4363	976
	PHARMACY PRACTICE	National Naval Med Ctr	ASHP	N	Bethesda	(301) 295-2115	340
	PHARMACY PRACTICE	Memorial Hosp at Easton, Maryland, Inc	ASHP	Y	Easton	(410) 822-1000	194
	PSYCHIATRY	Univ of Maryland	NO	N	Baltimore	(410) 706-1768	1380
	PSYCHIATRY	Univ of Maryland and Spring Grove Hosp Ctr	ASHP	N	Catonsville	(410) 363-2764	1293
Massachusetts	AMBULATORY/PRIMARY CARE	Beth Israel Hosp	NO	N	Boston	(617) 732-2825	1418
	HOME HEALTH CARE	Abbey Infusion Services	NO	N	Boston	(617) 732-9731	1020
	MANAGED CARE	Harvard Community Health Plan	NO	N	Boston	(617) 732-2875	1073
	PEDIATRICS	Children's Hospital	NO	N	Boston	(617) 355-5520	1461
	PHARMACY PRACTICE	Boston Med Ctr	NO	N	Boston	(617) 638-6789	1490
	PHARMACY PRACTICE	Boston Univ Med Ctr Hosp	ASHP	Y	Boston	(617) 638-6790	299
	PHARMACY PRACTICE	New England Med Ctr	ASHP	Y	Boston	(617) 636-5384	95
	PHARMACY PRACTICE	Harvard Pilgrim Health Care/Harvard Community Health	ASHP	Y	Boston	(617) 732-2875	1326
	PHARMACY PRACTICE	VA Med Ctr and Outpatient Clinics	ASHP	Y	Boston	(617) 278-4558	1406
	PHARMACY PRACTICE	Univ of Massachusetts Med Ctr	ASHP	Y	Worcester	(508) 856-2277	1371
Michigan	ADMINISTRATION	Detroit Receiving Hosp	ASHP	N	Detroit	(313) 745-4095	392
	COMMUNITY PHARMACY	Arbor Drugs Inc	NO	N	Detroit	(313) 577-5401	460
	CRITICAL CARE	Univ of MI	NO	N	Ann Arbor	(313) 763-9783	1436

Appendix E (cont.)

State or Province	Primary Focus	Site	Accred. Status	In ASHP Matching Program?	City	Contact Phone	RESFILE Record #
	CRITICAL CARE	Detroit Receiving Hosp & Univ Health Ctr	NO	N	Detroit	(313) 745-4550	1156
	GASTROENTEROLOGY	Univ of Michigan Med Ctr	NO	N	Ann Arbor	(313) 936-8210	1201
	HEMATOLOGY	Univ of Michigan Med Ctr	NO	N	Ann Arbor	(313) 936-8210	1202
	INFECTIOUS DISEASE	Univ of Michigan Med Ctr	NO	N	Ann Arbor	(313) 936-8210	1203
	INFECTIOUS DISEASE	Henry Ford Hosp	NO	N	Detroit	(313) 876-1799	1235
	INFECTIOUS DISEASE	Detroit Receiving Hosp	NO	N	Detroit	(313) 745-4554	287
	NEPHROLOGY	Univ of Michigan Med Ctr	NO	N	Ann Arbor	(313) 936-8210	831
	PEDIATRICS	Univ of MI Med Ctr Children's Hosp	NO	N	Ann Arbor	(313) 936-8985	1462
	PEDIATRICS	Univ of Michigan Med Ctr	NO	N	Ann Arbor	(313) 936-8210	830
	PHARMACOECONOMICS	St John Hosp and Med Ctr	NO	N	Detroit	(313) 343-3763	968
	PHARMACY PRACTICE	Univ of Michigan Hosp	ASHP	Y	Ann Arbor	(313) 936-8210	201
	PHARMACY PRACTICE	VA Med Ctr-Ann Arbor	ASHP	Y	Ann Arbor	(313) 769-7100	1397
	PHARMACY PRACTICE	Chelsea Community Hosp	NO	N	Chelsea	(313) 475-4010	344
	PHARMACY PRACTICE	Children's Hosp of Michigan	ASHP	Y	Detroit	(313) 745-5275	705
	PHARMACY PRACTICE	Harper Hosp	ASHP	Y	Detroit	(313) 745-9479	854
	PHARMACY PRACTICE	St John Hosp and Med Ctr	ASHP	Y	Detroit	(313) 343-3763	855
	PHARMACY PRACTICE	Grace Hosp	ASHP	Y	Detroit	(313) 966-3272	1328
	PHARMACY PRACTICE	Detroit Receiving Hosp/ Univ Health Ctr	ASHP	Y	Detroit	(313) 745-4554	381
	PHARMACY PRACTICE	Bronson Methodist Hosp	ASHP	Y	Kalamazoo	(616) 341-7999	12
	PHARMACY PRACTICE	Midmichigan Regional Med Ctr	ASHP	Y	Midland	(517) 839-1902	1407
	PHARMACY PRACTICE	William Beaumont Hosp	ASHP	Y	Royal Oak	(313) 551-4073	292
	PSYCHIATRY	Univ of Michigan Med Ctr	NO	N	Ann Arbor	(313) 936-8210	1205
	SURGERY	Univ of Michigan Med Ctr	NO	N	Ann Arbor	(313) 936-8210	1206
Minnesota	CRITICAL CARE	Mayo Med Ctr	NO	N	Rochester	(507) 255-7386	1432
	GERIATRICS	VA Med Ctr-Minneapolis	NO	N	Minneapolis	(612) 725-2040	491
	GERIATRICS	St. Paul-Ramsey Med Ctr	NO	N	St. Paul	(612) 221-8732	1439
	MANAGED CARE	Diversified Pharmaceutical Services	NO	N	Minneapolis	(612) 830-4117	1104
	NEPHROLOGY	Hennepin County Med Ctr	NO	N	Minneapolis	(612) 349-6348	424
	NEUROLOGY	MINCEP Epilepsy Care	NO	N	Minneapolis	(612) 525-2400	1250
	PEDIATRICS	Children's Health Care-St Paul	ASHP	N	St Paul	(612) 220-8877	681
	PHARMACY PRACTICE	VA Med Ctr-Minneapolis	ASHP	Y	Minneapolis	(612) 725-2040	767
	PHARMACY PRACTICE	Univ of Minnesota Hosp and Clinics	ASHP	Y	Minneapolis	(612) 626-3900	203
	PHARMACY PRACTICE	Hennepin County Med Ctr	ASHP	Y	Minneapolis	(612) 347-3217	1408
	PHARMACY PRACTICE	Abbott Northwestern Hosp	ASHP	Y	Minneapolis	(612) 863-4906	210
	PHARMACY PRACTICE	Mayo Med Ctr, Rochester/Methodist/St Mary's Hospitals	ASHP	Y	Rochester	(507) 255-5165	131
	PHARMACY PRACTICE	United and Children's Hosp	ASHP	Y	St Paul	(612) 220-8855	680
Mississippi	AMBULATORY/PRIMARY CARE	Univ of Mississippi Med Ctr	ASHP	N	Jackson	(601) 984-6834	1415
	FAMILY PRACTICE	Univ of Mississippi Med Ctr	NO	N	Jackson	(601) 984-6934	1438
	INFECTIOUS DISEASE	Univ of Mississippi Med Ctr	ASHP	N	Jackson	(601) 984-2617	575
	PEDIATRICS	Univ of Mississippi	ASHP	N	Jackson	(601) 984-2620	1261
	PHARMACY PRACTICE	Univ Hosp	ASHP	Y	Jackson	(601) 984-2055	329
	PHARMACY PRACTICE	North Mississippi Med Ctr	ASHP	Y	Tupelo	(601) 841-4361	1207

Appendix E (cont.)

State or Province	Primary Focus	Site	Accred. Status	In ASHP Matching Program?	City	Contact Phone	RESFILE Record #
Missouri	AMBULATORY/PRIMARY CARE	Veterans Affairs Med Ctr, John Cochran	ASHP	N	St Louis	(314) 652-4100	1172
	AMBULATORY/PRIMARY CARE	St Louis COP	NO	N	St Louis	(314) 367-8700	1421
	COMMUNITY PHARMACY	St Louis COP	NO	N	St Louis	(314) 367-8700	1422
	FAMILY PRACTICE	St John's Mercy Med Ctr	NO	N	St Louis	(314) 367-8700	1016
	GERIATRICS	VA Med Ctr-St Louis	ASHP	N	St Louis	(314) 894-6510	675
	INTERNAL MEDICINE	St Louis College of Pharmacy	NO	N	St Louis	(314) 367-8700	1244
	INTERNAL MEDICINE	Deaconess Hosp	NO	N	St Louis	(314) 367-8700	1173
	INTERNAL MEDICINE	St Louis COP	NO	N	St Louis	(314) 367-8700	1444
	MANAGED CARE	Group Health Plan of St Louis	NO	N	St Louis	(314) 367-8700	1248
	MANAGED CARE	Managed Prescription Services	NO	N	St Louis	(314) 259-4213	1247
	PEDIATRICS	Children's Mercy Hosp	NO	N	Kansas City	(816) 234-3024	1043
	PHARMACY PRACTICE	Harry S Truman Memorial Veterans Hosp	ASHP	Y	Columbia	(573) 443-2511	1409
	PHARMACY PRACTICE	VA Med Ctr-Kansas City, MO/Leavenworth, KS	ASHP	Y	Kansas City	(816) 861-4700	215
	PHARMACY PRACTICE	Cox Health Systems	ASHP	Y	Springfield	(417) 269-6286	1329
	PHARMACY PRACTICE	Dept of VA Med Ctr, John Cochran	ASHP	N	St Louis	(314) 289-6372	1331
	PHARMACY PRACTICE	St Louis Univ Hosp	ASHP	Y	St Louis	(314) 577-8067	998
	PHARMACY PRACTICE	Barnes and Jewish Hosp	ASHP	Y	St Louis	(314) 362-7714	9
	PSYCHIATRY	Western Missouri Mental Health Ctr	ASHP	N	Kansas City	(816) 512-4211	213
Nebraska	COMMUNITY PHARMACY	Travis Pharmacy, Shenandoah, Iowa	NO	N	Omaha	(402) 559-5366	1293
	COMPUTER TECHNOLOGY	Creighton Univ SOPAHP	NO	N	Omaha	(402) 280-3178	1295
	INTERNAL MEDICINE	Creighton Univ/St Joseph Hosp	NO	N	Omaha	(402) 280-2665	1475
	PHARMACOKINETICS	St Joseph Hosp	NO	N	Omaha	(402) 449-4572	438
	PHARMACY PRACTICE	Univ of Nebraska Hosp	ASHP	Y	Omaha	(402) 559-8253	219
Nevada	AMBULATORY/PRIMARY CARE	VA Med Ctr-Reno	NO	N	Reno	(702) 786-7200	1271
	PHARMACY PRACTICE	Univ Med Ctr	ASHP	Y	Las Vegas	(702) 383-2602	1332
	PHARMACY PRACTICE	Ioannis A Lougaris VAMC-Reno	ASHP	Y	Reno	(702) 328-1279	1333
	PHARMACY PRACTICE	Washoe Med Ctr	ASHP	Y	Reno	(702) 328-4753	867
New Jersey	DRUG INFORMATION	Roche Laboratories Inc	ASHP	N	Nutley	(201) 562-2395	880
	DRUG INFORMATION	Janssen Pharmaceutica	NO	N	Titusville	(800) 526-7736	1233
	EMERGENCY MEDICINE	Robert Wood Johnson Univ Hosp	NO	N	Piscataway	(908) 445-3285	134
	PHARMACY PRACTICE	St Barnabas Med Ctr	ASHP	Y	Livingston	(201) 533-5456	1334
	PHARMACY PRACTICE	Robert Wood Johnson Univ Hosp	ASHP	Y	New Brunswick	(908) 937-8582	330
	PHARMACY PRACTICE	The Med Ctr at Princeton	ASHP	Y	Princeton	(609) 497-4244	977
	PHARMACY PRACTICE	The Valley Hosp-Ridgewood	ASHP	Y	Ridgewood	(201) 447-8121	331
New Mexico	GERIATRICS	Senior Health Center	NO	N	Albuquerque	(505) 277-6333	1440
	PHARMACY PRACTICE	Presbyterian Healthcare Services	ASHP	Y	Albuquerque	(505) 841-1745	1410
	PHARMACY PRACTICE	VA Med Ctr-Albuquerque	ASHP	Y	Albuquerque	(505) 256-2757	271
New York	AMBULATORY/PRIMARY CARE	Stratton VA Med Ctr	NO	N	Albany	(518) 462-3311	1170
	AMBULATORY/PRIMARY CARE	VA Med Ctr	ASHP	N	Buffalo	(716) 834-9200	1486
	AMBULATORY/PRIMARY CARE	DVA Western NY Health Care System	NO	N	Buffalo	(716) 834-9200	1417
	AMBULATORY/PRIMARY CARE	Erie County Med Ctr	NO	N	Buffalo	(716) 898-4129	1004
	CRITICAL CARE	Maimonides Med Ctr	NO	N	Brooklyn	(718) 283-8031	1344

Appendix E (cont.)

State or Province	Primary Focus	Site	Accred. Status	In ASHP Matching Program?	City	Contact Phone	RESFILE Record #
	CRITICAL CARE	Maimonides Med Ctr	NO	N	Brooklyn	(718) 283-7207	1182
	GERIATRICS	Fay's Managed Pharmacy Service	NO	N	East Greenbush	(518) 479-0230	1483
	GERIATRICS	Monroe Community Hosp	NO	N	Rochester	(716) 274-7311	731
	INFECTIOUS DISEASE	Albany Med Ctr	NO	N	Albany	(518) 445-7209	906
	INFECTIOUS DISEASE	Millard Fillmore Health System	NO	N	Buffalo	(716) 887-4076	1389
	INFECTIOUS DISEASE	Bassett Healthcare	NO	N	Cooperstown	(607) 547-3399	1482
	INFECTIOUS DISEASE	Millard Fillmore Suburban Hosp	NO	N	Williamsville	(716) 568-3840	582
	NEPHROLOGY	Albany COP	NO	N	Albany	(518) 445-7235	1386
	NUTRITION	Albany Med Ctr	NO	N	Albany	(518) 445-7275	1387
	PHARMACY PRACTICE	Stratton VA Med Ctr	ASHP	Y	Albany	(518) 462-3311	700
	PHARMACY PRACTICE	St Peter's Hosp	NO	N	Albany	(518) 525-1266	893
	PHARMACY PRACTICE	Montefiore Med Ctr/Henry and Lucy Moss Division	ASHP	Y	Bronx	(718) 920-4529	497
	PHARMACY PRACTICE	VA Med Ctr-Bronx	ASHP	Y	Bronx	(718) 584-9000	1095
	PHARMACY PRACTICE	Brookdale Hosp Med Ctr	ASHP	Y	Brooklyn	(718) 240-5933	333
	PHARMACY PRACTICE	Erie County Med Ctr	NO	N	Buffalo	(716) 898-3284	29
	PHARMACY PRACTICE	The Buffalo General Hosp	ASHP	Y	Buffalo	(716) 845-2137	701
	PHARMACY PRACTICE	VA Med Ctr-Buffalo	NO	N	Buffalo	(716) 834-9200	1335
	PHARMACY PRACTICE	Bassett Healthcare	ASHP	Y	Cooperstown	(607) 547-3399	56
	PHARMACY PRACTICE	Fay's Managed Pharmacy Services	ASHP	Y	East Greenbush	(518) 479-0230	1336
	PHARMACY PRACTICE	The Mt Sinai Med Ctr	ASHP	Y	New York	(212) 241-6171	334
	PHARMACY PRACTICE	VA Med Ctr-New York	ASHP	Y	New York	(212) 686-7500	1337
	PHARMACY PRACTICE	Beth Israel Med Ctr	ASHP	Y	New York	(212) 420-2633	849
	PHARMACY PRACTICE	Veterans Affairs Med Ctr	ASHP	Y	Northport	(516) 261-4400	1411
	PHARMACY PRACTICE	Syracuse	NO	N	Syracuse	(315) 470-7412	1286
	PSYCHIATRY	Capital District Psychiatric Ctr	NO	N	Albany	(518) 445-7266	1055
North Carolina	DRUG INFORMATION	Campbell Univ SOP	ASHP	N	Buies Creek	(910) 893-1475	1287
	DRUG INFORMATION	Glaxo Wellcome, Inc	NO	N	Research Triangle Pk	(800) 334-0089	1479
	DRUG INFORMATION	Glaxo Wellcome Inc	NO	N	Research Triangle Pk	(800) 334-0089	576
	GERIATRICS	Univ of North Carolina at Chapel Hill	NO	N	Chapel Hill	(919) 962-0070	435
	GERIATRICS	Durham VA Med Ctr (182)	ASHP	N	Durham	(919) 286-6932	1219
	INFECTIOUS DISEASE	Univ of North Carolina at Chapel Hill	NO	N	Chapel Hill	(919) 962-0071	1241
	ONCOLOGY	Univ North Carolina Hosp	NO	N	Chapel Hill	(919) 962-0028	1457
	PEDIATRICS	Univ of North Carolina Hospitals	NO	N	Chapel Hill	(919) 966-6854	1463
	PHARMACOKINETICS	Univ of North Carolina Hosp	ASHP	N	Chapel Hill	(919) 966-6194	697
	PHARMACY PRACTICE	Mission and St Joe's Health System	ASHP	Y	Asheville	(704) 255-4354	1338
	PHARMACY PRACTICE	Univ of North Carolina Hospitals	ASHP	Y	Chapel Hill	(919) 966-5741	220
	PHARMACY PRACTICE	Univ of North Carolina Hospitals	ASHP	Y	Chapel Hill	(919) 962-0034	1208
	PHARMACY PRACTICE	Duke Univ Med Ctr	ASHP	Y	Durham	(919) 684-6353	618
	PHARMACY PRACTICE	Durham Regional Hosp	ASHP	Y	Durham	(919) 470-4342	609
	PHARMACY PRACTICE	VA Med Ctr-Durham	ASHP	Y	Durham	(919) 286-6959	1209
	PHARMACY PRACTICE	Moses H Cone Memorial Hosp	ASHP	Y	Greensboro	(910) 574-8124	91
	PHARMACY PRACTICE	Pitt County Memorial Hosp	ASHP	Y	Greenville	(919) 816-4481	980
	PHARMACY PRACTICE	Southeastern Regional Med Ctr	ASHP	Y	Lumberton	(910) 671-5175	997
	PHARMACY PRACTICE	Housecall Infusion Services	ASHP	Y	Raleigh	(919) 782-7488	1339

Appendix E (cont.)

State or Province	Primary Focus	Site	Accred. Status	In ASHP Matching Program?	City	Contact Phone	RESFILE Record #
	PHARMACY PRACTICE	North Carolina Baptist Hosp	ASHP	Y	Winston-Salem	(919) 716-6909	703
North Dakota	PHARMACY PRACTICE	St Alexius Med Ctr	ASHP	Y	Bismarck	(701) 224-7182	1340
	PHARMACY PRACTICE	VA Med Ctr-Fargo	ASHP	Y	Fargo	(701) 232-3241	1054
Ohio	ADMINISTRATION	Univ of Cincinnati Hosp	ASHP	N	Cincinnati	(513) 558-8803	165
	ADMINISTRATION	Riverside Methodist Hosp	ASHP	N	Columbus	(614) 566-5508	874
	AMBULATORY/PRIMARY CARE	Neighborhood Health Centers	NO	N	Columbus	(614) 292-2454	1094
	CARDIOLOGY	Ohio State Univ Med Ctr	NO	N	Columbus	(614) 293-8470	1426
	CRITICAL CARE	Univ of Cincinnati Hosp	ASHP	N	Cincinnati	(513) 558-5381	1012
	CRITICAL CARE	Cleveland Clinic Foundation	NO	N	Cleveland	(216) 444-1127	1485
	DRUG INFORMATION	Ohio State Univ Med Ctr	NO	N	Columbus	(614) 293-8470	1195
	GERIATRICS	VA Med Ctr-Cleveland	ASHP	N	Cleveland	(216) 791-3800	501
	INFECTIOUS DISEASE	Cleveland Clinic Foundation	NO	N	Cleveland	(216) 444-1127	1934
	INTERNAL MEDICINE	Ohio State University	NO	N	Columbus	(614) 292-5718	1442
	ONCOLOGY	Univ of Cincinnati Hosp	ASHP	N	Cincinnati	(513) 558-8808	164
	PEDIATRICS	Children's Hosp	ASHP	N	Columbus	(614) 722-2000	884
	PHARMACY PRACTICE	Univ of Cincinnati Hosp	ASHP	Y	Cincinnati	(513) 558-8808	163
	PHARMACY PRACTICE	Children's Hosp Med Ctr	ASHP	Y	Cincinnati	(513) 559-4862	16
	PHARMACY PRACTICE	VA Med Ctr-Cleveland	ASHP	Y	Cleveland	(216) 791-3800	274
	PHARMACY PRACTICE	Cleveland Clinic Foundation	NO	N	Cleveland	(216) 444-1127	1294
	PHARMACY PRACTICE	Mt Carmel Med Ctr	ASHP	Y	Columbus	(614) 234-1352	92
	PHARMACY PRACTICE	Riverside Methodist Hosp	ASHP	Y	Columbus	(614) 566-5508	661
	PHARMACY PRACTICE	Ohio State Univ Med Ctr	ASHP	Y	Columbus	(614) 293-8470	347
	PHARMACY PRACTICE	Grant/Riverside Methodist Hosp Grant Campus	ASHP	Y	Columbus	(614) 461-3417	32
	PHARMACY PRACTICE	Mt Carmel Med Ctr	ASHP	Y	Columbus	(614) 225-5830	1210
	PHARMACY PRACTICE	Ohio State Univ Med Ctr	ASHP	Y	Columbus	(614) 293-8470	807
	PHARMACY PRACTICE	Grant/Riverside Methodist Hosp Grant Campus	ASHP	Y	Columbus	(614) 461-3417	1159
	PHARMACY PRACTICE	Riverside Methodist Hosp	ASHP	Y	Columbus	(614) 566-5508	123
	PHARMACY PRACTICE	Lima Memorial Hosp	NO	N	Lima	(419) 226-5063	1263
	PHARMACY PRACTICE	The Toledo Hosp	NO	N	Toledo	(419) 471-5638	1150
	PSYCHIATRY	VA Med Ctr-Brecksville	NO	N	Brecksville	(216) 526-3030	1273
Oklahoma	AMBULATORY/PRIMARY CARE	Veterans Affairs Med Ctr/Dept of Pharm Practice and Univ of OK	ASHP	N	Oklahoma City	(405) 271-8000	812
	INFECTIOUS DISEASE	Univ of Oklahoma COP	NO	N	Oklahoma City	(405) 271-6878	1026
	INTERNAL MEDICINE	Univ of Oklahoma COP	NO	N	Oklahoma City	(405) 271-6878	1028
	ONCOLOGY	Univ of Oklahoma	NO	N	Oklahoma City	(405) 271-6878	1179
	PEDIATRICS	Children's Hosp of Oklahoma	NO	N	Oklahoma City	(405) 271-6878	1046
	PHARMACOKINETICS	VA Med Ctr-Oklahoma City	ASHP	N	Oklahoma City	(405) 270-1549	1217
	PHARMACOKINETICS	Univ of Oklahoma Health Sciences Ctr	NO	N	Oklahoma City	(405) 271-6878	923
	PHARMACY PRACTICE	Mercy Health Ctr	NO	N	Oklahoma City	(405) 752-3649	788
	PHARMACY PRACTICE	Integris Baptist Med Ctr	ASHP	Y	Oklahoma City	(405) 949-3068	8
	PHARMACY PRACTICE	WW Hastings Indian Hosp	ASHP	N	Tahlequah	(918) 458-3207	355
	PSYCHIATRY	VA Med Ctr-Oklahoma City	NO	N	Oklahoma City	(405) 270-0501	1347

Appendix E (cont.)

State or Province	Primary Focus	Site	Accred. Status	In ASHP Matching Program?	City	Contact Phone	RESFILE Record #
Oregon	AMBULATORY/PRIMARY CARE	VA Med Ctr	ASHP	N	Portland	(503) 220-8262	1487
	PHARMACY PRACTICE	VA Med Ctr-Portland	ASHP	Y	Portland	(503) 220-8262	276
	PHARMACY PRACTICE	Providence Med Ctr	ASHP	Y	Portland	(503) 215-6557	1211
	PHARMACY PRACTICE	Univ Hosp and Clinics-Portland	ASHP	Y	Portland	(503) 494-8007	112
Pennsylvania	ADMINISTRATION	Thomas Jefferson Univ Hosp	ASHP	N	Philadelphia	(215) 955-9055	390
	ADMINISTRATION	Pittsburgh Poison Ctr	NO	N	Pittsburgh	(412) 692-5600	119
	ADMINISTRATION	Univ of Pittsburgh Med Ctr	NO	N	Pittsburgh	(412) 647-5926	873
	AMBULATORY/PRIMARY CARE	Univ of Pittsburgh Med Ctr	NO	N	Pittsburgh	(412) 647-3309	1312
	CRITICAL CARE	Hamot Med Ctr	ASHP	N	Erie	(814) 877-6021	652
	CRITICAL CARE	Hosp of the Univ of Pennsylvania	NO	N	Philadelphia	(215) 596-8582	1391
	CRITICAL CARE	Univ of Pennsylvania Med Ctr	NO	N	Philadelphia	(215) 895-1159	1392
	CRITICAL CARE	Hosp of the Univ of Pennsylvania	NO	N	Philadelphia	(215) 596-8854	446
	CRITICAL CARE	Allegheny General Hosp	ASHP	N	Pittsburgh	(412) 359-6630	1402
	CRITICAL CARE	Univ of Pittsburgh Med Ctr	NO	N	Pittsburgh	(412) 647-5943	754
	DRUG INFORMATION	Temple Univ Hosp	ASHP	N	Philadelphia	(215) 707-4643	821
	DRUG INFORMATION	Thomas Jefferson Univ Hosp	ASHP	N	Philadelphia	(215) 955-9055	401
	DRUG INFORMATION	Univ of Pittsburgh Med Ctr	NO	N	Pittsburgh	(412) 624-5214	634
	INFECTIOUS DISEASE	Temple Univ Hosp	NO	N	Philadelphia	(215) 707-4643	1178
	MANAGED CARE	HealthAmerica Pharmacy	NO	N	Pittsburgh	(412) 577-4368	1445
	MANAGED CARE	Stadlanders Managed Pharmacy Services	NO	N	Pittsburgh	(412) 825-8331	1447
	NEPHROLOGY	Univ of Pittsburgh Med Ctr	NO	N	Pittsburgh	(412) 624-8153	1310
	NEUROLOGY	Germantown Hospital and Med Ctr	NO	N	Philadelphia	(215) 951-8035	1451
	NUTRITION	Temple Univ Hosp	NO	N	Philadelphia	(215) 707-4643	1035
	ONCOLOGY	Philadelphia VA Med Ctr	NO	N	Philadelphia	(215) 596-8874	1255
	ONCOLOGY	Univ of Pittsburgh Med Ctr	ASHP	N	Pittsburgh	(412) 624-3417	882
	PEDIATRICS	Philadelphia CPS	NO	N	Philadelphia	(215) 596-8889	1393
	PHARMACOKINETICS	Thomas Jefferson Univ Hosp	NO	N	Philadelphia	(215) 955-9055	508
	PHARMACY PRACTICE	Lehigh Valley Hosp	NO	N	Allentown	(215) 402-8880	608
	PHARMACY PRACTICE	Hamot Med Ctr	ASHP	Y	Erie	(814) 877-2526	34
	PHARMACY PRACTICE	Univ Hosp/Hershey Med Ctr/Penn State Univ	ASHP	Y	Hershey	(717) 531-6378	507
	PHARMACY PRACTICE	Suburban General Hosp	ASHP	Y	Norristown	(215) 278-2125	336
	PHARMACY PRACTICE	Thomas Jefferson Univ Hosp	ASHP	Y	Philadelphia	(215) 955-9055	149
	PHARMACY PRACTICE	Hosp of the Univ of Pennsylvania	ASHP	Y	Philadelphia	(215) 662-2900	226
	PHARMACY PRACTICE	Temple Univ Hosp	ASHP	Y	Philadelphia	(215) 707-4525	148
	PHARMACY PRACTICE	VA Med Ctr-Pittsburgh	ASHP	Y	Pittsburgh	(412) 692-3380	1394
	PHARMACY PRACTICE	Allegheny General Hosp	ASHP	Y	Pittsburgh	(412) 359-3500	7
	PHARMACY PRACTICE	Univ of Pittsburgh Med Ctr	ASHP	Y	Pittsburgh	(412) 647-8270	850
Rhode Island	AMBULATORY/PRIMARY CARE	VA Med Ctr-Providence	ASHP	N	Providence	(401) 457-3048	1220
	INFECTIOUS DISEASE	URI Roger Williams Med Ctr	NO	N	Providence	(401) 456-2261	228
South Carolina	AMBULATORY/PRIMARY CARE	Med Univ of South Carolina	NO	N	Charleston	(803) 792-8564	1419
	AMBULATORY/PRIMARY CARE	Charleston VA Med Ctr	NO	N	Charleston	(803) 577-5011	1416
	AMBULATORY/PRIMARY CARE	Richland Memorial Hosp	NO	N	Columbia	(803) 434-7245	1226
	CRITICAL CARE	Med Univ of South Carolina	ASHP	N	Charleston	(803) 792-2663	71

Appendix E (cont.)

State or Province	Primary Focus	Site	Accred. Status	In ASHP Matching Program?	City	Contact Phone	RESFILE Record #
	DRUG INFORMATION	Med Univ of South Carolina	ASHP	N	Charleston	(803) 792-7527	73
	FAMILY PRACTICE	Med Univ of South Carolina	NO	N	Charleston	(803) 792-6427	1075
	INTERNAL MEDICINE	Med Univ of South Carolina	ASHP	N	Charleston	(803) 792-5537	74
	INTERNAL MEDICINE	Dorn Veterans Hosp	NO	N	Columbia	(803) 777-7888	1396
	MANAGED CARE	Med Univ of South Carolina	NO	N	Charleston	(803) 792-3606	1289
	NUCLEAR PHARMACY	Med Univ of South Carolina	ASHP	N	Charleston	(803) 792-7458	667
	ONCOLOGY	Richland Memorial Hosp	NO	N	Columbia	(803) 434-7254	819
	PEDIATRICS	Med Univ of South Carolina Children's Hosp	ASHP	N	Charleston	(803) 792-7524	76
	PEDIATRICS	Richland Memorial Hosp	NO	N	Columbia	(803) 434-7245	412
	PHARMACOTHERAPY	Med Univ of South Carolina	NO	N	Charleston	(803) 792-7628	1472
	PHARMACY PRACTICE	Med Univ of South Carolina	ASHP	Y	Charleston	(803) 792-2665	593
	PHARMACY PRACTICE	Richland Memorial Hosp	ASHP	Y	Columbia	(803) 434-7254	130
	PSYCHIATRY	Med Univ of South Carolina	ASHP	N	Charleston	(803) 792-0182	77
South Dakota	PEDIATRICS	Sioux Valley Hosp	NO	N	Sioux Falls	(605) 333-7362	1259
	PHARMACY PRACTICE	McKennan Hosp	ASHP	Y	Sioux Falls	(605) 333-8872	1305
Tennessee	CARDIOLOGY	Memphis VA Med Ctr	NO	N	Memphis	(901) 448-4869	1397
	COMMUNITY PHARMACY	Univ of Tennessee COP	NO	N	Nashville	(615) 256-3023	649
	CRITICAL CARE	Baptist Memorial Hosp	NO	N	Memphis	(901) 448-7197	1309
	CRITICAL CARE	Regional Med Ctr at Memphis	NO	N	Memphis	(901) 448-6513	238
	GERIATRICS	VA Med Ctr-Memphis	NO	N	Memphis	(901) 577-7363	1090
	HOME HEALTH CARE	Medical Alternatives	NO	N	Millington	(800) 872-2209	1021
	NUTRITION	Univ of Tennessee Med Ctr at Knoxville	ASHP	Y	Knoxville	(615) 544-9134	1306
	PEDIATRICS	Le Bonheur Children's Med Ctr	NO	N	Memphis	(901) 448-7145	237
	PHARMACOKINETICS	St Jude Children's Research Hosp	NO	N	Memphis	(901) 522-0663	1267
	PHARMACY PRACTICE	Erlanger Med Ctr	ASHP	Y	Chattanooga	(423) 778-5063	1412
	PHARMACY PRACTICE	Univ of Tennessee Med Ctr at Knoxville	ASHP	Y	Knoxville	(615) 544-9124	805
	PHARMACY PRACTICE	VA Med Ctr-Memphis	ASHP	Y	Memphis	(901) 523-8990	596
	PHARMACY PRACTICE	Regional Med Ctr at Memphis	ASHP	Y	Memphis	(901) 545-7847	383
	PHARMACY PRACTICE	Baptist Memorial Hosp	ASHP	Y	Memphis	(901) 227-4358	1086
	PHARMACY PRACTICE	St Jude Children's Research Hosp	NO	N	Memphis	(901) 522-0660	1089
	PHARMACY PRACTICE	Methodist Hosp of Memphis	ASHP	Y	Memphis	(901) 726-8445	765
	PHARMACY PRACTICE	VA Med Ctr-Nashville	ASHP	Y	Nashville	(615) 327-4751	859
	PHARMACY PRACTICE	Vanderbilt Univ Hosp	ASHP	Y	Nashville	(615) 322-2374	982
	PHARMACY PRACTICE	St Thomas Hosp	ASHP	N	Nashville	(615) 222-6708	778
	PSYCHIATRY	Memphis Mental Health Inst	NO	N	Memphis	(901) 528-6044	232
	TRANSPLANTATION	Univ of Tennessee Bowld Hosp	NO	N	Memphis	(901) 448-4136	1277
Texas	AMBULATORY/PRIMARY CARE	Scott & White Hosp	NO	N	Austin	(817) 724-7458	1424
	AMBULATORY/PRIMARY CARE	Audie L Murphy Memorial Veterans' Hosp	ASHP	N	San Antonio	(512) 617-5139	239
	CRITICAL CARE	Hermann Hosp	ASHP	N	Houston	(713) 704-1559	896
	CRITICAL CARE	Texas Southern Univ-The Methodist Hosp	ASHP	N	Houston	(713) 313-7570	985
	CRITICAL CARE	Scott & White Hosp	NO	N	Temple	(817) 724-1731	1314
	DRUG INFORMATION	Scott & White Hosp	NO	N	Temple	(817) 774-3811	597
	GERIATRICS	Audie Murphy Mermorial VAMC-San Antonio	ASHP	N	San Antonio	(210) 617-5215	240

Appendix E (cont.)

State or Province	Primary Focus	Site	Accred. Status	In ASHP Matching Program?	City	Contact Phone	RESFILE Record #
	INFECTIOUS DISEASE	Audie L Murphy Memorial Veterans Hosp	ASHP	N	San Antonio	(210) 617-5138	247
	INTERNAL MEDICINE	Univ of Texas COP	NO	N	Austin	(512) 471-4048	1030
	INTERNAL MEDICINE	Univ of Texas Health Science Ctr	NO	N	San Antonio	(210) 567-8355	1245
	INTERNAL MEDICINE	Scott & White Hosp	NO	N	Temple	(817) 724-4636	1243
	MANAGED CARE	Texas Dept of Criminal Justice	NO	N	Huntsville	(409) 291-6896	1448
	NUTRITION	St Mary of the Plains Hosp	ASHP	N	Lubbock	(806) 796-6776	1253
	NUTRITION	Audie L Murphy Memorial Veterans Hosp	ASHP	N	San Antonio	(210) 617-5300	244
	ONCOLOGY	University of TX, MD Anderson Cancer Ctr	ASHP	N	Houston	(713) 792-2870	625
	ONCOLOGY	Audie L Murphy Memorial Veterans' Hosp	ASHP	N	San Antonio	(210) 617-5300	241
	ONCOLOGY	Univ of Texas Health Science Ctr	NO	N	San Antonio	(210) 567-8339	1257
	ONCOLOGY	Scott & White Hosp	NO	N	Temple	(817) 724-1731	1454
	PEDIATRICS	Children's Med Ctr of Dallas	ASHP	N	Dallas	(214) 640-2398	1398
	PEDIATRICS	Hermann Hosp	NO	N	Houston	(713) 797-2070	1003
	PHARMACY PRACTICE	High Plains Baptist Hosp	ASHP	Y	Amarillo	(806) 356-2234	718
	PHARMACY PRACTICE	Baylor Univ Med Ctr	ASHP	Y	Dallas	(214) 820-2114	612
	PHARMACY PRACTICE	Parkland Memorial Hosp	ASHP	Y	Dallas	(214) 590-8714	356
	PHARMACY PRACTICE	Veterans Affairs Med Ctr	ASHP	Y	Dallas	(214) 376-5451	1413
	PHARMACY PRACTICE	Univ of Texas Med Branch at Galveston	ASHP	Y	Galveston	(409) 772-1174	357
	PHARMACY PRACTICE	Methodist Hosp	ASHP	Y	Houston	(713) 790-2141	525
	PHARMACY PRACTICE	Hermann Hosp	ASHP	Y	Houston	(713) 704-2070	986
	PHARMACY PRACTICE	Owen Healthcare Inc	ASHP	Y	Houston	(713) 777-8173	987
	PHARMACY PRACTICE	St Luke's Episcopal Hosp	ASHP	Y	Houston	(713) 791-3114	716
	PHARMACY PRACTICE	Univ of Houston/COP/Texas Dept of Criminal Justice	ASHP	Y	Huntsville	(409) 291-6896	1212
	PHARMACY PRACTICE	Wilford Hall Med Ctr	ASHP	N	Lackland AFB	(210) 670-5416	1213
	PHARMACY PRACTICE	Southwest Texas Methodist Hosp	ASHP	Y	San Antonio	(210) 593-6942	984
	PHARMACY PRACTICE	Scott & White Hosp	NO	N	Temple	(817)724-5287	1492
	PHARMACY PRACTICE	Scott & White Hosp	NO	N	Temple	(817) 724-5287	1491
	PSYCHIATRY	Univ of Texas at Austin/Austin State Hosp	NO	N	Austin	(512) 419-2757	1282
	PSYCHIATRY	Univ of Texas Health Science Ctr at San Antonio	ASHP	N	San Antonio	(210) 567-8355	624
	TRANSPLANTATION	Hermann Hosp	NO	N	Houston	(713) 704-2070	1275
Utah	DRUG INFORMATION	Univ of Utah Hosp and Clinics	ASHP	N	Salt Lake City	(801) 581-2073	249
	PHARMACY PRACTICE	VA Med Ctr-Salt Lake City	ASHP	Y	Salt Lake City	(801) 582-1565	1000
	PHARMACY PRACTICE	Univ of Utah Hospitals & Clinics	ASHP	Y	Salt Lake City	(801) 581-2189	664
Vermont	PHARMACY PRACTICE	Med Ctr Hosp of Vermont	ASHP	Y	Burlington	(802) 656-2885	300
Virginia	AMBULATORY/PRIMARY CARE	Med College of Virginia Hosp	ASHP	N	Richmond	(804) 828-0215	65
	AMBULATORY/PRIMARY CARE	McGuire VA Med Ctr	NO	N	Richmond	(804) 675-5292	1070
	ASSOCIATION MANAGEMENT	American Society of Consultant Pharmacists	NO	N	Alexandria	(703) 739-1300	98
	COMMUNITY PHARMACY	Richmond Medication Consultants	NO	N	Richmond	(804) 359-1395	1431
	CRITICAL CARE	Med College of Virginia Hosp	NO	N	Richmond	(804) 828-0215	470
	DRUG INFORMATION	Med College of Virginia Hosp	NO	N	Richmond	(804) 828-0215	66
	GERIATRICS	McGuire VA Med Ctr	NO	N	Richmond	(804) 230-1422	1154
	INTERNAL MEDICINE	McGuire VA Med Ctr	NO	N	Richmond	(804) 230-1422	1027
	ONCOLOGY	Med College of Virginia	NO	N	Richmond	(804) 828-6098	1254

Appendix E (cont.)

State or Province	Primary Focus	Site	Accred. Status	In ASHP Matching Program?	City	Contact Phone	RESFILE Record #
	ONCOLOGY	Medical Coll of Virginia Hospitals	NO	N	Richmond	(804) 828-0215	1299
	PHARMACY PRACTICE	Univ of Virginia Health Sciences Ctr	ASHP	y	Charlottesville	(804) 924-2910	853
	PHARMACY PRACTICE	Fairfax Hosp	ASHP	y	Falls Church	(703) 698-3734	610
	PHARMACY PRACTICE	John Randolph Med Ctr	ASHP	y	Hopewell	(804) 458-6650	342
	PHARMACY PRACTICE	Med Coll of Virginia Hosp	ASHP	y	Richmond	(804) 828-0215	852
	PHARMACY PRACTICE	VA Med Ctr-Salem	ASHP	y	Salem	(703) 982-2463	1214
Washington	ADMINISTRATION	St Joseph Med Ctr	ASHP	N	Tacoma	(206) 591-6692	395
	AMBULATORY/PRIMARY CARE	Virginia Mason Med Ctr	NO	N	Monroe	(360) 794-5555	227
	AMBULATORY/PRIMARY CARE	Family Med Ctr, Univ of WA Med Ctr	ASHP	N	Seattle	(206) 548-5618	251
	AMBULATORY/PRIMARY CARE	Univ of WA Med Ctr/Harborview Med Ctr	NO	N	Seattle	(206) 548-6060	1423
	AMBULATORY/PRIMARY CARE	Virginia Mason Med Ctr	NO	N	Seattle	(206) 583-6011	1227
	DRUG INFORMATION	Washington State Univ	NO	N	Spokane	(509) 358-7665	604
	MANAGED CARE	Virginia Mason Med Ctr	NO	N	Seattle	(206) 583-6011	1449
	ONCOLOGY	Univ of WA Med Ctr/Harborview Med Ctr	NO	N	Seattle	(206) 548-6060	250
	PHARMACY PRACTICE	Overlake Hosp Med Ctr	ASHP	y	Bellevue	(206) 688-5059	722
	PHARMACY PRACTICE	Good Samaritan Hosp	ASHP	y	Puyallup	(206) 841-5899	994
	PHARMACY PRACTICE	Franciscan Home Infusion	ASHP	y	Redmond	(206) 885-5544	1341
	PHARMACY PRACTICE	Valley Med Ctr	ASHP	y	Renton	(206) 251-5188	616
	PHARMACY PRACTICE	Group Health Coop of Puget Sound Ctrl Hosp	ASHP	y	Seattle	(206) 443-4388	660
	PHARMACY PRACTICE	VA Med Ctr-Seattle	ASHP	y	Seattle	(206) 764-2142	283
	PHARMACY PRACTICE	Univ of Washington Med Ctr/Harborview Med Ctr	ASHP	y	Seattle	(206) 548-6060	1480
	PHARMACY PRACTICE	Sacred Heart Med Ctr	ASHP	y	Spokane	(509) 626-4569	721
	PHARMACY PRACTICE	St Joseph Med Ctr	ASHP	y	Tacoma	(206) 591-6692	780
	PHARMACY PRACTICE	Madigan Arrmy Med Ctr	ASHP	N	Tacoma	(206) 968-2015	1489
	PHARMACY PRACTICE	Southwest Washington Med Ctr	NO	N	Vancouver	(360) 256-3034	1493
	PSYCHIATRY	Washington State Univ	NO	N	Spokane	(509) 299-4348	1274
West Virginia	CRITICAL CARE	Charleston Area Med Ctr	ASHP	N	Charleston	(304) 348-3926	1232
	PHARMACOTHERAPY	Charleston Area Med Ctr	ASHP	N	Charleston	(304) 348-6283	1304
	PHARMACY PRACTICE	Charleston Area Med Ctr	ASHP	y	Charleston	(304) 348-6283	704
	PHARMACY PRACTICE	VA Med Ctr-Huntington	ASHP	y	Huntington	(304) 429-6755	981
	PHARMACY PRACTICE	West Virginia Univ Hosp	ASHP	y	Morgantown	(304) 598-4148	291
	TRANSPLANTATION	West Virginia Univ Hosp	NO	N	Morgantown	(304) 598-4148	1298
Wisconsin	ADMINISTRATION	Univ of Wisconsin Hosp and Clinics	ASHP	N	Madison	(608) 263-1290	255
	AMBULATORY/PRIMARY CARE	William S Middleton VA Hosp	ASHP	N	Madison	(608) 262-7077	284
	PHARMACY PRACTICE	Mercy Hosp	ASHP	y	Janesville	(608) 756-6846	1215
	PHARMACY PRACTICE	Meriter Hosp	ASHP	y	Madison	(608) 267-6160	87
	PHARMACY PRACTICE	Univ of Wisconsin Hosp and Clinics	ASHP	y	Madison	(608) 263-1290	253
	PHARMACY PRACTICE	St Luke's Med Ctr	ASHP	y	Milwaukee	(414) 649-7931	1342
	PHARMACY PRACTICE	Froedtert Memorial Lutheran Hosp	ASHP	y	Milwaukee	(414) 259-2991	1216
	PHARMACY PRACTICE	Clement J Zablocki VA Med Ctr	ASHP	y	Milwaukee	(414) 384-2000	1343

Appendix E (cont.)

State or Province	Primary Focus	Site	Accred. Status	In ASHP Matching Program?	City	Contact Phone	RESFILE Record #
CANADA							
Alberta	GENERAL HOSPITAL	Calgary General Hosp	CaSHP	N	Calgary	(403) 268-9175	1114
	GENERAL HOSPITAL	Alberta Children's Hosp	CaSHP	N	Calgary	(403) 229-7939	1113
	GENERAL HOSPITAL	Royal Alexandra Hosp	CaSHP	N	Edmonton	(403) 477-4460	1181
	GENERAL HOSPITAL	Caritas Health Group	CaSHP	N	Edmonton	(403) 450-7411	1115
	GENERAL HOSPITAL	Univ of Alberta Hosp	CaSHP	N	Edmonton	(403) 492-6988	1116
British Columbia	GENERAL HOSPITAL	Burnaby Hosp	CaSHP	N	Burnaby	(604) 431-4742	1108
	GENERAL HOSPITAL	Royal Inland Hosp	CaSHP	N	Kamloops	(604) 374-5111	1283
	GENERAL HOSPITAL	Royal Columbian Hosp	CaSHP	N	New Westminister	(604) 520-4259	539
	GENERAL HOSPITAL	Lions Gate Hosp	CaSHP	N	North Vancouver	(604) 984-5919	905
	GENERAL HOSPITAL	British Columbia Children's Hosp	CaSHP	N	Vancouver	(604) 8752710	1109
	GENERAL HOSPITAL	Vancouver Hosp & Health Sciences Ctr	CaSHP	N	Vancouver	(604) 875-4077	1112
	GENERAL HOSPITAL	St Paul's Hosp	CaSHP	N	Vancouver	(604) 682-2344	1111
	PSYCHIATRY	Riverview Hosp	NO	N	Port Coquitlam	(604) 524-7210	933
Manitoba	GENERAL HOSPITAL	Misericordia Gen Hosp	NO	N	Winnipeg	(204) 788-8239	1122
	GENERAL HOSPITAL	Health Sciences Centre	CaSHP	N	Winnipeg	(204) 787-1232	1121
Nova Scotia	GENERAL HOSPITAL	Camp Hill Medical Ctr	CaSHP	N	Halifax	(902) 496-4393	1146
	GENERAL HOSPITAL	Victoria General Hosp	CaSHP	N	Halifax	(902) 428-3579	1147
Ontario	DRUG INFORMATION	Ottawa Gen Hosp/Glaxo Canada Inc	NO	N	Ottawa	(613) 737-8344	1155
	GENERAL HOSPITAL	Chedoke-McMaster Hosp	CaSHP	N	Hamilton	(416) 521-2100	1124
	GENERAL HOSPITAL	Henderson Hosp	NO	N	Hamilton	(905) 389-4411	1317
	GENERAL HOSPITAL	St Joseph's Hosp	CaSHP	N	Hamilton	(905) 522-1155	1129
	GENERAL HOSPITAL	Kingston General Hosp	CaSHP	N	Kingston	(613) 548-6021	1166
	GENERAL HOSPITAL	Victoria Hosp	CaSHP	N	London	(519) 667-6584	1133
	GENERAL HOSPITAL	Ottawa Civic Hosp	CaSHP	N	Ottawa	(613) 761-4154	1127
	GENERAL HOSPITAL	Ottawa General Hosp	CaSHP	N	Ottawa	(613) 737-8344	1128
	GENERAL HOSPITAL	Wellesley Hosp	CaSHP	N	Toronto	(416) 926-4840	1494
	GENERAL HOSPITAL	Sunnybrook Health Science Ctr	CaSHP	N	Toronto	(416) 480-6100	1132
	GENERAL HOSPITAL	The Wellesley Hosp	CaSHP	N	Toronto	(416) 926-4840	1134
	GENERAL HOSPITAL	Addiction Research Foundation	CaSHP	N	Toronto	(416) 595-6560	1123
	GENERAL HOSPITAL	The Toronto Hosp	CaSHP	N	Toronto	(416) 603-5800	1131
	GENERAL HOSPITAL	St Michael's Hosp	CaSHP	N	Toronto	(416) 864-5702	1130
	GENERAL HOSPITAL	Hosp for Sick Children	CaSHP	N	Toronto	(416) 813-6475	708
	GENERAL HOSPITAL	Mt Sinai Hosp	CaSHP	N	Toronto	(416) 586-5016	1126
	GENERAL HOSPITAL	Women's College Hosp	CaSHP	N	Toronto	(416) 586-8420	1135
	NUCLEAR PHARMACY	Chedoke-McMaster Hosp	NO	N	Hamilton	(905) 521-2100	1315
	NUCLEAR PHARMACY	Toronto Hosp	NO	N	Toronto	(416) 603-5800	1316
Québec	GENERAL HOSPITAL	C H Cite de la Sante de Laval	CaSHP	N	Laval	(514) 662-5503	1136
	GENERAL HOSPITAL	Hopital Notre-Dame	CaSHP	N	Montreal	(514) 876-6844	1138
	GENERAL HOSPITAL	C H Saint Luc	CaSHP	N	Montreal	(514) 281-6163	1137
	GENERAL HOSPITAL	C H du Sacre-Coeur	CaSHP	N	Montreal	(514) 338-2666	1140

Appendix E (cont.)

State or Province	Primary Focus	Site	Accred. Status	In ASHP Matching Program?	City	Contact Phone	RESFILE Record #
	GENERAL HOSPITAL	C H Sainte-Justine	CaSHP	N	Montreal	(514) 345-4603	1141
	GENERAL HOSPITAL	Hopital Royal Victoria	CaSHP	N	Montreal	(514) 843-1601	1142
	GENERAL HOSPITAL	C H General Juif	CaSHP	N	Montreal	(514) 340-7504	1143
	GENERAL HOSPITAL	C H General de Montreal	CaSHP	N	Montreal	(514) 937-6011	1144
	GENERAL HOSPITAL	CH Universitaire de Sherbrooke	CaSHP	N	Sherbrooke	(819) 563-5555	1284
	GENERAL HOSPITAL	C H Hotel Dieu de Sherbrooke	CaSHP	N	Sherbrooke	(819) 822-6725	1145
	GENERAL HOSPITAL	C H St-Joseph de Trois-Rivieres	CaSHP	N	Trois-Rivieres	(819) 372-3560	1139
	INFECTIOUS DISEASE	Univ of Montreal	NO	N	Montreal	(514) 343-2052	1350
Saskatchewan	GENERAL HOSPITAL	Regina Health District	CaSHP	N	Regina	(306) 766-2317	1119
	GENERAL HOSPITAL	St Paul's Hosp	CaSHP	N	Saskatoon	(306) 664-5060	1117
	GENERAL HOSPITAL	Saskatoon City Hosp	CaSHP	N	Saskatoon	(306) 664-5060	1118
	GENERAL HOSPITAL	Royal Univ Hosp	CaSHP	N	Saskatoon	(306) 966-5060	1120

APhA COMMUNITY PHARMACY RESIDENCIES*

Title	Eligibility/Description	Award	Deadline	Information
University of the Pacific Community Pharmacy Residency Program	Graduates of accredited US pharmacy schools and foreign pharmacy graduates certified by FPGEC; licensed or immediately eligible for licensure following graduation.	Stipend varies with program; low $20k's	Varies	Katherine Knapp University of the Pacific School of Pharmacy Stockton, CA 95211 (209) 946-2594
University of Kansas Community Pharmacy Residency Program	Graduates of accredited US pharmacy schools and foreign pharmacy graduates certified by FPGEC; licensed or immediately eligible for licensure following graduation.	Stipend varies with program; low $20k's	Varies	University of Kansas Harold N. Godwin, Chair Pharmacy Practice Medical Center 3901 Rainbow Blvd. Kansas City, KS 66160 (913) 588-2330
University of Maryland at Baltimore Community Pharmacy Residency Program	Graduates of accredited US pharmacy schools and foreign pharmacy graduates certified by FPGEC; licensed or immediately eligible for licensure following graduation.	Stipend varies with program; low $20k's	Varies	University of MD at Baltimore Stuart T. Haines, PharmD, BCPS, CDE Dept. of Pharmacy Practice & Science 506 West Fayette St., Rm. 203 Baltimore, MD 21201-1715 (410) 706-1865
Wayne State University Community Pharmacy Residency Program	Graduates of accredited US pharmacy schools and foreign pharmacy graduates certified by FPGEC; licensed or immediately eligible for licensure following graduation.	Stipend varies with program; low $20k's	Varies	Wayne State University Geralynn Smith, Residency Director College of Pharmacy 328 Shapero Hall Detroit, MI 48202 (313) 577-5401

Appendix E (cont.)

Title	Eligibility/Description	Award	Deadline	Information
University of Nebraska Community Pharmacy Residency Program	Graduates of accredited US pharmacy schools and foreign pharmacy graduates certified by FPGEC; licensed or immediately eligible for licensure following graduation.	Stipend varies with program; low $20k's	Varies	University of NE Medical Center Warren Narducci, PharmD Residency Directory Dept. of Pharmacy Practice UNMC College of Pharmacy 600 South 42nd Street Omaha, NE 68198-6045 (402) 559-5366
North Dakota State University Community Pharmacy Residency Program	Graduates of accredited US pharmacy schools and foreign pharmacy graduates certified by FPGEC; licensed or immediately eligible for licensure following graduation.	Stipend varies with program; low $20k's	Varies	North Dakota State University Harvey J. Hanel, PharmD College of Pharmacy Fargo, ND 58105 (701) 231-8801
Ohio State University Community Pharmacy Residency Program	Graduates of accredited US pharmacy schools and foreign pharmacy graduates certified by FPGEC; licensed or immediately eligible for licensure following graduation.	Stipend varies with program; low $20k's	Varies	The Ohio State University Gerald L. Cable College of Pharmacy 500 West 12th Avenue Columbus, OH 43210-1291 (614) 292-2492
University of Pittsburgh Community Pharmacy Residency Program	Graduates of accredited US pharmacy schools and foreign pharmacy graduates certified by FPGEC; licensed or immediately eligible for licensure following graduation.	Stipend varies with program; low $20k's	Varies	University of Pittsburgh Grace Lamsam, PharmD, PhD College of Pharmacy 904 Salk Hall Pittsburgh, PA 15261 (412) 648-7192
Medical University of South Carolina Community Pharmacy Residency Program	Graduates of accredited US pharmacy schools and foreign pharmacy graduates certified by FPGEC; licensed or immediately eligible for licensure following graduation.	Stipend varies with program; low $20k's	Varies	Medical University of South Carolina C.W. Weart, PharmD College of Pharmacy 171 Ashley Avenue Charleston, SC 29425 (803) 792-3606
University of Tennessee Community Pharmacy Residency Program	Graduates of accredited US pharmacy schools and foreign pharmacy graduates certified by FPGEC; licensed or immediately eligible for licensure following graduation.	Stipend varies with program; low $20k's	Varies	University of Tennessee Roger Davis, PharmD College of Pharmacy Dept. of Clinical Pharmacy 26 S. Dunlap, Room 202 Memphis, TN 38163 (901) 448-6041 or (615) 256-3023
Medical College of Virginia/VCU Community Pharmacy Residency Program	Graduates of accredited US pharmacy schools and foreign pharmacy graduates certified by FPGEC; licensed or immediately eligible for licensure following graduation.	Stipend varies with program; low $20k's	Varies	Medical College of Virginia/VCU Ralph Small, PharmD Residency Director School of Pharmacy 410 N. 12th Street - Smith Bldg. Richmond, VA 23298-0533 (410) 542-2500

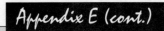

Title	Eligibility/Description	Award	Deadline	Information
University of Washington Community Pharmacy Residency Program	Graduates of accredited US pharmacy schools and foreign pharmacy graduates certified by FPGEC; licensed or immediately eligible for licensure following graduation.	Stipend varies with program; low $20k's	Varies	University of Washington Terri O'Sullivan Residency Director School of Pharmacy Box 357631 Seattle, WA 98195 (206) 543-3324

*Source: Interorganizational Council on Student Affairs, Interorganizational Financial and Experiential Information Document, July 18, 1996.
Several, but not all, of these programs are included in RESFILE 97.

Appendix F

RESFILE 97 Fellowships

State or Province	Primary Focus	Site	City	Contact Phone	RESFILE Record #
USA					
Arizona	PHARMACOECONOMICS	Univ of Arizona COP	Tucson	(602) 626-5730	1048
Arkansas	CARDIOLOGY	Univ Hosp of Arkansas	Little Rock	(501) 686-6393	1231
California	INFECTIOUS DISEASE	Univ of Southern California	Los Angeles	(213) 342-3434	231
	INFECTIOUS DISEASE	Univ of California, San Francisco	San Francisco	(415) 476-1927	541
	INFECTIOUS DISEASE	St Zion Med Ctr of UCSF	San Francisco	(415) 885-7468	1237
	NEUROLOGY	Univ of California, San Francisco	San Francisco	(415) 476-5587	1033
	PHARMACOECONOMICS	Kaiser Permanente	Downey	(310) 803-2937	1465
	PHARMACOECONOMICS	USC	Los Angeles	(213) 342-1474	1279
Colorado	AMBULATORY/PRIMARY CARE	Univ of Colorado	Denver	(303) 270-5229	1353
	PHARMACOKINETICS	National Jewish Ctr for Immunology & Respiratory Medicine	Denver	(303) 398-1427	1264
Connecticut	CARDIOLOGY	Hartford Hosp	Hartford	(203) 545-2221	312
	INFECTIOUS DISEASE	Hartford Hosp	Hartford	(203) 545-2865	311
	PHARMACOECONOMICS	Hartford Hosp	Hartford	(860) 545-2865	1464
	PHARMACOECONOMICS	Hartford Hosp	Hartford	(203) 545-2221	1290
	PHARMACY PRACTICE	Hartford Hosp	Hartford	(203) 545-2912	971
Florida	BIOTECHNOLOGY	VA Med Ctr-Bay Pines	Bay Pines	(813) 398-9431	1229
	CARDIOLOGY	Univ of Florida COP	Gainesville	(904) 392-3155	912
	PULMONARY CARE	Univ of Florida	Gainesville	(904) 392-5677	1358
Georgia	CARDIOLOGY	Univ of GA	Augusta	(706) 721-3994	1429
	CRITICAL CARE	Med Coll of Georgia	Augusta	(706) 721-4915	552
Idaho	SUBSTANCE ABUSE	Idaho State Univ/Boise VA Hosp	Boise	(208) 386-0989	1308
Illinois	CARDIOLOGY	Univ of Illinois, Chicago	Chicago	(312) 996-3267	674
	CARDIOLOGY	Univ of Illinois	Chicago	(312) 413-7594	1364
	CLINICAL PHARMACOLOGY	Univ of Illinois Coll of Medicine at Peoria	Peoria	(309) 671-3412	1266
	INFECTIOUS DISEASE	Univ of Illinois Hosp/Michael Reese Hosp	Chicago	(312) 996-0892	673
	INFECTIOUS DISEASE	Univ of Illinois	Chicago	(312) 996-8639	1365
	INFECTIOUS DISEASE	Univ of IL at Peoria	Peoria	(309) 671-8403	1481
	NEUROLOGY	Univ of Illinois Hosp/Michael Reese Hosp	Chicago	(312) 996-5549	840
	ONCOLOGY	Univ of Illinois	Chicago	(312) 996-0886	1366
	PHARMACOECONOMICS	Univ Hosp Consortium	Oak Brook	(708) 954-1700	936
Indiana	PHARMACOECONOMICS	Purdue Univ	West Lafayette	(317) 494-1468	1278

Appendix F (cont.)

State or Province	Primary Focus	Site	City	Contact Phone	RESFILE Record #
Iowa	CARDIOLOGY	Univ of IA	Iowa City	(319) 335-8752	1430
	INFECTIOUS DISEASE	Univ of Iowa	Iowa City	(319) 335-8861	1360
	PHARMACOKINETICS	Univ of Iowa COP	Iowa City	(319) 335-8804	926
	PSYCHIATRY	Univ of Iowa	Iowa City	(319) 335-8803	1361
	RHEUMATOLOGY	Univ of Iowa	Iowa City	(319) 353-8877	1474
	TRANSPLANTATION	Univ of Iowa COP	Iowa City	(319) 338-8839	1061
Kentucky	CARDIOLOGY	Univ of Kentucky Med Ctr	Lexington	(606) 233-5085	325
	DRUG RESEARCH	Univ of Kentucky	Lexington	(606) 257-3321	560
	PHARMACOKINETICS	Univ of Kentucky Med Ctr	Lexington	(606) 257-3378	324
	PSYCHIATRY	Eastern State Psychiatric Hosp	Lexington	(606) 246-7449	1369
Maryland	GERIATRICS	Varies	Bethesda	(301) 657-3000	1184
	ONCOLOGY	National Cancer Institute	Bethesda	(301) 402-3622	1039
	PHARMACOKINETICS	Univ of Maryland	Baltimore	(410) 706-7338	1378
	PSYCHIATRY	Varies	Bethesda	(301) 657-3000	1185
Michigan	CARDIOLOGY	Henry Ford Hosp	Detroit	(313) 876-3458	1230
	CRITICAL CARE	Univ of MI	Ann Arbor	(313) 763-9783	1435
	CRITICAL CARE	Henry Ford Hosp	Detroit	(313) 876-1234	39
	INFECTIOUS DISEASE	Detroit Receiving Hosp	Detroit	(313) 745-4554	1382
	PHARMACOECONOMICS	Detroit Receiving Hosp	Detroit	(313) 745-4025	1297
	PHARMACOKINETICS	Wayne State Univ	Detroit	(313) 577-8899	566
Minnesota	CARDIOLOGY	St Paul-Ramsey Med Ctr	St Paul	(612) 221-3482	1428
	GERIATRICS	Hennepin County Med Ctr	Minneapolis	(612) 347-5618	432
	INFECTIOUS DISEASE	Univ of Minnesota COP	Minneapolis	(612) 624-6489	431
	INFECTIOUS DISEASE	St Paul-Ramsey Med Ctr	St Paul	(612) 221-3896	569
	PEDIATRICS	Children's Health Care-Minneapolis	Minneapolis	(612) 863-6906	567
	PHARMACOKINETICS	Hennepin County Med Ctr	Minneapolis	(612) 347-6367	1049
	PULMONARY CARE	Allergy and Asthma Specialists, PA	Minneapolis	(612) 333-2200	1058
	TRANSPLANTATION	Hennepin County Med Ctr	Minneapolis	(612) 347-6367	422
	TRANSPLANTATION	Abbott Northwestern Hosp/MPLS Heart Institute Foundation	Minneapolis	(612) 863-3620	751
Mississippi	INFECTIOUS DISEASE	Univ of Mississippi Med Ctr	Jackson	(601) 984-2621	909
Missouri	BIOTECHNOLOGY	Washington Univ Med Ctr	St Louis	(314) 367-8700	574
	DRUG RESEARCH	Deaconess Hosp	St Louis	(314) 367-8700	903
Nebraska	CARDIOLOGY	Creighton Univ Cardiac Ctr	Omaha	(402) 280-4288	439
	CRITICAL CARE	Univ of Nebraska Med Ctr	Omaha	(402) 559-9016	1383
New Jersey	DRUG RESEARCH	Rutgers Univ	Piscataway	(908) 932-3285	133
	MANAGED CARE	Janssen Pharmaceuticals	Titusville	(609) 730-3044	1458
	NEUROLOGY	Rutgers Univ	Piscataway	(908) 828-3000	1452
	PHARMACOECONOMICS	Sandoz Pharmaceuticals Corp	East Hanover	(201) 503-7241	1385
	PHARMACOECONOMICS	Bristol-Myers Squibb	Princeton	(609) 897-2741	1384
	PHARMACOECONOMICS	Ciba Pharmaceuticals Division	Summit	(908) 277-5367	1186

Appendix F (cont.)

State or Province	Primary Focus	Site	City	Contact Phone	RESFILE Record #
New York	CARDIOLOGY	Millard Fillmore Hosp	Buffalo	(716) 887-4704	1008
	CLINICAL PHARMACOLOGY	Bassett Healthcare	Cooperstown	(607) 547-3399	1148
	DRUG RESEARCH	Millard Fillmore Health System	Buffalo	(716) 887-4917	1388
	INFECTIOUS DISEASE	SUNY at Buffalo	Amhearst	(716) 645-3635	583
	NEPHROLOGY	Albany Med Ctr	Albany	(512) 445-7235	737
	PHARMACOECONOMICS	Pharmaceutical Outcomes Research Inc	Williamsville	(716) 633-6463	1262
	PHARMACOKINETICS	SUNY at Buffalo	Buffalo	(716) 633-3463	1265
	PHARMACOKINETICS	Millard Fillmore Health System	Buffalo	(716) 887-4917	1390
	PHARMACOKINETICS	Pharmaceutical Outcomes Research, Inc	Williamsville	(716) 633-3463	1471
North Carolina	CARDIOLOGY	Univ of North Carolina, Chapel Hill	Chapel Hill	(919) 962-0072	578
	DRUG RESEARCH	Univ of North Carolina, Chapel Hill	Chapel Hill	(919) 962-0072	1013
	GERIATRICS	Duke Univ Medical Center	Durham	(919) 681-8777	1484
	GERIATRICS	East Carolina Univ	Greenville	(919) 816-3838	434
	PEDIATRICS	Greensboro AHEC	Greensboro	(910) 574-7570	1031
	PHARMACOECONOMICS	Glaxo Wellcome Inc	Research Triangle Pk	(919) 483-3525	436
	PHARMACOKINETICS	Univ of North Carolina, Chapel Hill SOP/Glaxo Wellcome	Chapel Hill	(919) 962-7030	225
Ohio	BIOTECHNOLOGY	Ohio State Univ	Columbus	(614) 292-0075	1228
	CARDIOLOGY	Ohio State Univ	Columbus	(614) 292-7103	106
	CRITICAL CARE	Ohio State Univ	Columbus	(614) 292-6352	108
	INFECTIOUS DISEASE	Ohio State Univ Med Ctr	Columbus	(614) 292-2416	1193
	INFECTIOUS DISEASE	Children's Hosp	Columbus	(614) 722-2880	105
	LONG TERM CARE	Ohio State Univ	Columbus	(614) 292-9713	1459
	NEUROLOGY	Ohio State Univ Coll of Pharmacy	Columbus	(614) 292-9713	1251
	PHARMACOECONOMICS	Ohio State Univ/Glaxo Wellcome	Columbus	(614) 292-6415	1466
Oklahoma	CARDIOLOGY	Univ of Oklahoma Health Science Ctr	Oklahoma City	(405) 271-6878	892
	PHARMACOKINETICS	Univ of Oklahoma	Oklahoma City	(405) 271-6878	1280
Pennsylvania	CARDIOLOGY	Philadelphia COP & Science	Philadelphia	(215) 895-1152	1009
	CARDIOLOGY	Hosp of the Univ of Pennsylvania	Philadelphia	(215) 596-8576	645
	CRITICAL CARE	Hosp of the Univ of Pennsylvania	Philadelphia	(215) 596-8854	1011
	NEPHROLOGY	Univ of Pittsburgh	Pittsburgh	(412) 624-8153	738
	ONCOLOGY	Philadelphia COP & Science	Philadelphia	(215) 596-8831	512
	PHARMACOECONOMICS	Thomas Jefferson Univ/SmithKline Beecham	Philadelphia	(215) 955-1159	1469
	PHARMACOECONOMICS	Thomas Jefferson Univ	Philadelphia	(215) 955-1159	1468
	PHARMACOECONOMICS	Thomas Jefferson Univ/Janssen Pharmaceutica	Philadelphia	(215) 955-1159	1467
	SAFE MEDICATION MANAGEMENT	The Ctr for Proper Medication Use	Philadelphia	(215) 895-1131	942
	SAFE MEDICATION MANAGEMENT	Institute for Safe Medication Practices	Warminster	(215) 956-9181	1313
	TRANSPLANTATION	Univ of Pittsburgh	Pittsburgh	(412) 648-8559	1276
Rhode Island	CARDIOLOGY	Univ of Rhode Island	Kingston	(401) 792-2734	1395
South Carolina	INFECTIOUS DISEASE	Med Univ of South Carolina	Charleston	(803) 792-8501	1236
Tennessee	CARDIOLOGY	Univ of Tennessee	Memphis	(901) 528-6041	595
	CRITICAL CARE	Univ of Tennessee	Memphis	(901) 448-6470	1037

Appendix F (cont.)

State or Province	Primary Focus	Site	City	Contact Phone	RESFILE Record #
	CRITICAL CARE	Regional Med Ctr at Memphis	Memphis	(901) 448-6041	234
	INFECTIOUS DISEASE	Univ of Tennessee	Memphis	(901) 448-6041	236
	NUTRITION	Univ of Tennessee	Memphis	(901) 528-6420	1038
	ONCOLOGY	St Jude Children's Research Hosp	Memphis	(901) 495-2348	594
	PEDIATRICS	Le Bonheur Children's Med Ctr	Memphis	(901) 448-7145	1092
	PHARMACOKINETICS	St Jude Children's Research Hosp	Memphis	(901) 522-0663	1268
	PHARMACOKINETICS	St Jude Children's Research Hosp	Memphis	(901) 522-0663	144
	PHARMACOKINETICS	St Jude Children's Research Hosp	Memphis	(901) 495-3665	677
	TECHNOLOGY	VA Med Ctr-Murfreesboro	Murfreesboro	(615) 893-1360	1097
Texas	DRUG RESEARCH	Univ of Texas Health Science Ctr	San Antonio	(512) 567-8339	900
	GERIATRICS	Univ of Houston	Houston	(714) 795-8378	1399
	INTERNAL MEDICINE	Univ of Texas Health Science Ctr	San Antonio	(210) 567-8355	1246
	PHARMACOKINETICS	Univ of Texas Health Science Ctr	San Antonio	(210) 567-8355	1400
	PSYCHIATRY	Univ of Texas at Austin	Austin	(512) 471-4048	1272
	PSYCHIATRY	Univ of Texas Health Science Ctr	San Antonio	(210) 567-8355	242
Utah	CARDIOLOGY	Univ of Utah	Salt Lake City	(801) 581-6165	890
Virginia	INFECTIOUS DISEASE	Med Coll of Virginia	Richmond	(804) 828-8317	603
	PHARMACOECONOMICS	ASCP Research & Education Foundation	Alexandria	(703) 739-1300	1291
	RHEUMATOLOGY	Med College of Virginia Hosp	Richmond	(804) 828-6333	69
Washington	INFECTIOUS DISEASE	Deaconess Med Ctr	Spokane	(509) 358-7658	910
	PHARMACOECONOMICS	Univ of Washington	Seattle	(206) 685-8153	1470
	PHARMACOKINETICS	Univ of Washington	Seattle	(206) 685-2713	252
	PSYCHIATRY	VA PSHCS Med Ctr	Seattle	(206) 764-2142	1152
Wisconsin	NEPHROLOGY	Univ of Wisconsin Hosp and Hazleton Laboratories	Madison	(608) 263-5536	607
	ONCOLOGY	Univ of Wisconsin Comprehensive Cancer Ctr	Madison	(608) 263-2496	254
	PHARMACOECONOMICS	Univ of Wisconsin Hosp and Clinics	Madison	(608) 262-7537	1401
CANADA					
British Columbia	INFECTIOUS DISEASE	Vancouver Hosp & Health Sciences Ctr	Vancouver	(604) 875-4077	1171
	PHARMACEUTICAL CARE	Univ of British Columbia	Vancouver	(604) 822-2343	1478
Manitoba	INFECTIOUS DISEASE	Univ of Manitoba	Winnipeg	(204) 787-4902	1240
Ontario	PHARMACOKINETICS	Sunnybrook Health Science Centre	Toronto	(416) 480-4508	522
Québec	CARDIOLOGY	Hospital de Sacre-Coeur de Montreal	Montreal	(514) 338-2506	1349
	PHARMACOKINETICS	Univ of Montreal	Montreal	(514) 343-2052	1351

Appendix G

Pharmacy Residencies and Fellowships: A Time Line for Preparation and Exploration

Preprofessional or Early Professional Years

1. Explore the career options available to pharmacists.
2. Become involved in extracurricular professional and service activities that are of interest to you.
3. Consider doing at least one independent study research project during your academic years.
4. Do an internship or volunteer at one or more pharmacy practice sites to obtain internship hours and gain practice experience.
5. Attend one or more APhA Annual Meetings. Network with other students and practitioners and attend forums on postgraduate educational options.

Fall/Winter before Next-to-Last Year of Undergraduate Training (or earlier)

1. Start identifying your short-term (less than five years) and long-term professional goals.
2. Acquire basic information about residencies and fellowships.
3. Discuss residencies, fellowships, and other options with your adviser or a faculty member who has completed a residency or fellowship.
4. Learn as much as you can about practice areas of interest; for example, ask to "shadow" a practitioner or clinical faculty member for a few hours.
5. Consider presenting the findings of your independent research at local, regional, or national forums, or submit a manuscript for publication.

Spring/Summer before Last Year of School

1. Talk with graduating students who have applied for residencies or fellowships.
2. Look through the RESFILE and residency and fellowship directories. Start screening programs for desired location, focus, or other characteristics.
3. Plan to attend the ASHP Midyear Clinical Meeting and schedule some interviews.

Fall of Last Year of School

1. Use the newest edition of RESFILE to again screen for target programs of interest.
2. Using RESFILE, generate letters to program contacts to request further information and application materials.
3. Review the materials and send letters to programs in which you are interested, requesting an interview at the ASHP Midyear Clinical Meeting. (Remember, however, that on-campus interviews are usually also required and desirable.)
4. If you are thinking about a general pharmacy practice residency, consider signing up for the ASHP Resident Matching Program by late September. This ensures that you will get a personal copy of the *Residency Directory* when it is published in October.
5. Sign up for the Personnel Placement Service at the ASHP Midyear Clinical Meeting. Some programs conduct preliminary residency and fellowship candidate interviews there. Sign up before the deadline to save money!
6. Check the ASHP and ACCP directories for additional information on programs of interest.
7. Create a curriculum vitae or résumé.

Appendix G (cont.)

Winter of Last Year of School

1. Attend the ASHP Midyear Clinical Meeting in December and talk with representatives of programs in which you are interested. Set realistic limits (e.g., fewer than 10 programs). Browse at the Residency Showcase.
2. Immediately after the Midyear, send thank you letters to programs in which you are still interested and confirm your intention to apply.
3. Prepare applications to the programs you have chosen (limit it to six). Observe the deadlines. Remember that you must apply to each program directly, regardless of whether you intend to participate in the Resident Matching Program.
4. Begin scheduling interviews. Try to group two or three in the same area. If you intend to participate in the ASHP Resident Matching Program, you must complete these interviews before the program's mid-January deadline.
5. If you are considering participation in the Resident Matching Program, submit your initial application materials before the mid-January deadline.

Spring of Last Year of School

1. If you have decided to participate in the Resident Matching Program, submit your match choice list by the early March deadline.
2. If you are also considering nonaccredited or nonmatching (but accredited) specialty residencies, decide whether you are going to commit to the program early and not submit a match choice list in March. Or, if you do not obtain a position in the match, you may contact nonaccredited programs or those accredited programs that did not fill all their positions once the matching process is completed. ASHP will provide a list of accredited residencies with positions still available.
3. If you participated in the accredited pharmacy practice Resident Matching Program, you will be informed of the results in late March. Most accredited and nonaccredited residencies and fellowships begin on July 1.

Appendix H

Sample RESFILE Program Record

RECORD #: 1295
Information current as of 10/01/96
Academic Affiliation: Creighton Univ SOPAHP
Site: Creighton Univ SOPAHP
Program Available Since: 1995
Contact: Dr. Wayne Young, Pharm.D., 2500 California Plaza, Omaha, NE 68178
Phone: (402) 280-3178 Ext:
Residency/Fellowship: Residency
Primary Focus: Computer Technology
Additonal Program Emphases: Pharmacocybernetics Drug Information
Other Programs are available at this site.
Accreditation: N ASHP Match: N
ACCP Directory: N ASHP Directory: N
Stipend: $24,000 - $26,000
Number of Positions Offered: 1
Duration of Program (years): 1
On-site Interview Required: N
Application Deadline: NI Start Date: July 1
Academic Course Work: optional Academic degree: N
U.S./Canadian (as applicable) Citizenship Required: Y
In-State/Province License Required: N
Health Insurance: Y Sick Leave: Y Vacation: Y Meeting Benefit: Y

Comments: The Pharmacy Informatics Residency is a postgraduate training program that prepares pharmacists for leadership roles in developing and maintaining pharmacy-related computer information systems. The residency is a twelve-month training experience based in the computer laboratories and drug information centers of the School of Pharmacy and Allied Health Professions. The resident will have experiences in developing and supervising various student computing systems and operations in all three of the School's student computer laboratories. The School's three computing laboratories have more than 60 Windows PCs, five different file servers, and full Internet access and functionality. The resident will work directly with the residency director in managing these computing environments and will work on a specific project during the residency program. To improve their teaching skills the resident will assist the residency director in preparing and giving presentations in several information management courses created for Doctor of Pharmacy students. The resident will also have three one-month rotations in the School's drug information service units. During these rotations the resident will participate in all aspects of the teaching and service activities of the centers. However, the resident's training will focus on information management systems that support the operation of the respective centers with particular emphasis placed on remote connectivity and computer-based communication systems that assist all the centers to share information and resources.

Appendix I

Sample Inquiry Letter Generated by RESFILE

John Doe
1200 N. Applebee Street
Orchard, IA 51500
(712) 211-4343

December 6, 1996

Warren Narducci, Pharm.D.
University of Nebraska Medical Center
College of Pharmacy
600 S. 42nd St.
Omaha, NE 68198-6045

Re: Residency
At: Travis Community Pharmacy
With primary focus in: Community Pharmacy

Dear Dr. Narducci:

I am a pharmacy student at the University of Iowa Medical Center. I am interested in doing a residency with a focus in community practice. Your program is one that appears perfect to enable me to pursue my future professional goals. Would you please send me information and application materials about your program?

I am looking forward to hearing from you.

Sincerely,

John Doe

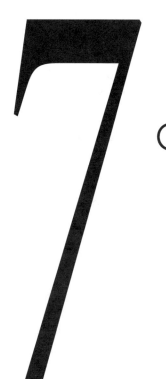

Chapter 7

Getting Your License

Introduction

Before you can practice pharmacy in the United States, you must become licensed. To continue to practice, you must renew your license each year. This requires successful completion of a certain number of continuing-education units (CEUs). The licensure process is regulated at the state level and coordinated by the National Association of Boards of Pharmacy (NABP).

This chapter explains the role of state boards of pharmacy and provides an overview of what you'll need to do to get licensed and relicensed. A special section contains information needed by graduates of foreign pharmacy schools.

State Boards of Pharmacy

There are 64 boards of pharmacy across the United States, Canada, Puerto Rico, the Virgin Islands, and Australia. State boards of pharmacy operate under the authority of their state legislature.

Each board has an executive director (or secretary), several elected members (usually around seven), and a cadre of inspectors who travel the state. The inspectors visit pharmacies to help them comply with state regulations and investigate complaints that have been filed against pharmacists. The elected members include both pharmacists and lay people. Board members promulgate uniform standards of practice throughout the state, examine candidates for licensure, oversee the relicensure process, and discipline those responsible for violating state pharmacy practice acts. A directory of the state boards of pharmacy in the United States appears as Appendix J.

Getting Licensed

To become a registered pharmacist, you must fulfill both national and state requirements.

NAPLEX™

Candidates for licensure must pass the North American Pharmacist Licensure Examination, or NAPLEX™. NAPLEX is developed by NABP for administration by the state boards of pharmacy. It is used in all states except California, which has its own test. State examination requirements are summarized in Appendix K.

NAPLEX is a computer-adaptive test that assesses the candidate's ability to apply knowledge gained in pharmacy school to practice situations. The examination consists of 150 multiple-choice questions, many of which refer to information provided in a patient profile. Half of the questions concern managing drug therapy to optimize patient outcome, about one fourth focus on ensuring the safe and accurate preparation and dispensing of medications, and the remainder cover providing drug information and promoting public health. The questions are written by practitioners, educators, and regulators from across the country.

NAPLEX is given four times a year. Application forms are available from NABP. The examination fee, which must be paid at the time of application, is $250.

Drug Law Examinations

When you take the NAPLEX, you will also take two pharmacy law examinations: the Federal Drug Law Examination (FDLE®) and a state law examination. The FDLE consists of 70 multiple-choice questions. State examinations vary in length and cover state-specific statutes.

Laboratory Examinations

Some states require that licensure candidates pass a laboratory examination. The purpose of this test is to ensure that candidates can accurately and safely prepare and dispense medications.

Check with your state board of pharmacy to determine whether this is required in the state in which you seek licensure.

Internships

All state boards of pharmacy require candidates to complete an internship before licensure (Appendix L). Internships usually consist of 1,500 hours of experience that are gained during pharmacy school (beginning after you have completed your first year of training). Some states require that internship hours be gained solely after graduation from pharmacy school and before licensure.

The internship process is subject to state board regulations. Each intern, internship site, and preceptor must register with the state board of pharmacy to have the hours counted toward licensure.

Relicensure

Forty-nine state boards of pharmacy require (or will soon require) pharmacists to complete a certain number of CEUs before they can renew their licenses each year. CEUs must be secured through a program approved by the American Council on Pharmaceutical Education (ACPE). Details about CEU requirements in each state are provided in Appendix M.

Most states require pharmacists to acquire approximately

15 hours of continuing education annually. ACPE-approved CEUs may be secured through articles that appear in professional journals, local seminars and regional, state, and national meetings, home study certificate courses, videotapes and audiotapes, and teleconferences.

To document completion of a continuing-education experience, the pharmacist must take a multiple-choice examination that is submitted to the provider. A score of 75%–80% is generally required to pass. Candidates who pass receive a certificate from the provider. The certificate must be turned in to the state board as verification of the number of CEUs completed.

Score and Licensure Transfer

If you wish to transfer a NAPLEX score to more than one state, the request must be submitted at the time you register to take the exam. If you sit for the FDLE in certain participating states, you may transfer your score to states in which you wish to hold an additional license by completing NABP's FDLE Score Transfer Form. Score transfer fees apply.

The licensure transfer process can be time consuming. If you plan to relocate, start early. Requirements for transferring pharmacy licensure from one state to another are summarized in Appendix N.

"Oath of a Pharmacist"

The "Oath of a Pharmacist" is taken by all new pharmacists upon graduation. A copy of the oath, along with a brief interpretation, follows.

The "Oath of a Pharmacist" is based on the "Oath and Prayer of Maimonides" with input from the American Pharmaceutical Association (APhA) and the American Association of Colleges of Pharmacy (AACP). The AACP Board of Directors approved the oath in 1983 and has made it available to every college and school of pharmacy.

The characteristics of a professional pharmacy practitioner are described in the oath such that we obtain an understanding of the meaning of the word "professional." Professionals devote their lives to a significant social value. Pharmacy is a

Oath of a Pharmacist

At this time, I vow to devote my professional life to the service of all humankind through the profession of pharmacy.

I will consider the welfare of humanity and relief of human suffering my primary concerns.

I will apply my knowledge, experience, and skills to the best of my ability to assure optimal drug therapy outcomes for the patients I serve.

I will keep abreast of developments and maintain professional competency in my profession of pharmacy.

I will maintain the highest principles of moral, ethical, and legal conduct.

I will embrace and advocate change in the profession of pharmacy that improves patient care.

I take these vows voluntarily with the full realization of the responsibility with which I am entrusted by the public.

Developed by the American Pharmaceutical Association Academy of Students of Pharmacy and the American Association of Colleges of Pharmacy Council of Deans Task Force on Professionalism, June 26, 1994.

learned profession requiring individuals to dedicate themselves voluntarily to acquiring and maintaining exceptional knowledge and skills to provide pharmaceutical care within an ethical context.

The first two statements of the oath describe a commitment to the service of humankind, the welfare of humanity, and the relief of human suffering as the pharmacist's primary concerns. Further, these statements emphasize that this commitment is lifelong in nature and should be practiced without discrimination. Specifically, the concept of pharmaceutical care embraces a covenantal relationship with the patient and other health care providers to ensure that optimal therapeutic outcomes are attained.

The next two statements accentuate the character of a pharmacist in exceeding the knowledge and skills of all others in providing pharmaceutical care and services to the public and other health professionals. A lifetime of learning in pharmacy is necessary to maintain one's professional stature and to provide the services inherent to the profession. The acquisition of knowledge and skills by pharmacists must serve to advance the profession. Professional competency involves participation in organizations that support and speak for the profession. Pharmacists promote unity within the profession and enthusiastically accept the responsibilities and accountability for membership in the profession.

The fifth statement characterizes the pharmacist's commitment to live a life characterized by faithfulness to high moral principles and ethical conduct. This is manifested not only in abiding by and enforcing the laws governing the practice of pharmacy but also in ensuring that the laws support the primary mission of the profession, the delivery of pharmaceutical care. Pharmacists must exhibit moral and ethical conduct in their daily interactions with patients and other health care providers. Pharmacists dedicate themselves to excellence in their knowledge, skill, and caring because they adhere to high moral and ethical principles. This enables them to maintain a covenantal relationship with society.

The next statement describes pharmacy as a profession where change must be embraced, rather than resisted. Pharmacists must actively participate as agents of change, focusing on improving health care.

The last statement of the oath describes the pharmacist as voluntarily making these vows with full understanding of the responsibility they impose.

Professionalism requires constant attention. The seeds of professionalism are sown when students begin their preparation for pharmacy school, are cultivated and nurtured in pharmacy school, and are brought to fruition and maintained during their careers as pharmacists. Becoming a professional means more than learning the science of pharmacy. It means mastering the art of pharmaceutical care in service to fellow human beings. This service must be carried out with dignity, integrity, and honor as reflected in this oath.

Information for Foreign Pharmacy Graduates

The Foreign Pharmacy Graduate Examination Committee (FPGEC), which is part of NABP, defines a "foreign pharmacy graduate" as a pharmacist whose undergraduate pharmacy degree was conferred by a recognized school of pharmacy outside the 50 United States, the District of Columbia, and

Puerto Rico. Recognized schools of pharmacy are those colleges and universities listed in the World Health Organization's *World Directory of Schools of Pharmacy* or otherwise approved by the FPGEC. United States citizens who have completed their pharmacy education outside the United States are, therefore, considered to be "foreign pharmacy graduates," whereas foreign nationals who have graduated from schools in the United States are not.

If a foreign graduate's pharmacy school is not listed in the *World Directory of Schools of Pharmacy*, the FPGEC considers applications from such graduates on a case-by-case basis.

FPGEC Licensure Process

If you are a foreign pharmacy graduate who wishes to practice pharmacy in the United States, you must be licensed by the state in which you wish to practice. To be licensed by a state board of pharmacy, you must meet the educational, experiential, and other requirements of the state in addition to passing the licensure examinations that are administered by that state.

Essential information about state requirements is summarized here. Be sure to contact the board of pharmacy of the state(s) in which you are interested to learn exactly what is required of foreign pharmacy graduates.

Age

To be licensed as a pharmacist, you must be:
• 18 years old in California, Connecticut, District of Columbia, Florida, Georgia, Indiana, Kentucky, Maryland, Massachusetts, Michigan, New Hampshire, North Carolina, North Dakota, Ohio, Oregon, Rhode Island, South Dakota, Tennessee, Texas, Vermont, Virginia, Washington, and West Virginia
• 19 years old in Alabama
• 21 years old in Arkansas, Colorado, Delaware, Illinois, Louisiana, Maine, Minnesota, Missouri, Nebraska, New Jersey, New York, Pennsylvania, and Puerto Rico.
• Of legal age in Iowa and Kansas. Check with the state board to determine the exact age requirement.
• Age of majority in Idaho, New Mexico, Wyoming, and Hawaii. Check with the state board to determine the exact age requirement.
• Alaska, Arizona, Mississippi, Montana, Nevada, Oklahoma, South Carolina, Utah, and Wisconsin have no age requirements.

Citizenship

Full United States citizenship is required for licensure in Maine.

Citizenship, legal declaration of intention, or resident alien status is required in Louisiana, New Jersey, New York, and Hawaii.

Applicants are individually reviewed by the board in Kentucky.

Meeting Educational Eligibility Requirements

To be licensed, a pharmacist must have graduated from a school of pharmacy approved by a state board of pharmacy or accredited by the American Council on Pharmaceutical Education (ACPE). Except for the School of Pharmacy at the University of Puerto Rico, no school of pharmacy outside the United States holds ACPE accreditation.

Graduates of foreign pharmacy schools may meet the educational eligibility requirements for licensure by
• Graduating from a U.S. school or college of pharmacy;
• Earning FPGEC certification; and/or
• Following other procedures approved by the state in which licensure is sought.

Graduation from a U.S. College or School of Pharmacy

Advance standing, based on credentials and transcripts, may be awarded to foreign gradu-

99

ates. Apply to the dean of the college in which you are interested. If you graduated from a U.S. school of pharmacy and fulfill other requirements, you will be eligible to take licensure examinations.

FPGEC Certification

To obtain an FPGEC certificate, you must pass the Foreign Pharmacy Graduate Equivalency Examination (FPGEE) and obtain a score of a least 550 on the Test of English as a Foreign Language (TOEFL).

FPGEE

To be accepted to take the FPGEE, you must have obtained a degree or qualification from a school of pharmacy program that had at least a four-year curriculum leading to pharmacy license or its equivalent.

For more information, write to the FPGEC, National Association of Boards of Pharmacy, 700 Busse Highway, Park Ridge, Illinois 60068.

TOEFL

For FPGEC certification, you must obtain a score of at least 550 on the TOEFL. States that do not participate in the FPGEC certification program may also have requirements for demonstrating English language proficiency. They may have additional requirements, such as the Test of Spoken English (TSE) or other tests of English language proficiency. Check with the appropriate state board to determine these requirements.

For more information about the TOEFL, contact TOEFL Services, P.O. Box 6151, Princeton, NJ 08541-6151. Telephone (609) 951-1100.

State-Specific Requirements

The following states have requirements beyond those of the FPGEC. Before applying for FPGEC certification, check with the board of pharmacy of the state in which you are seeking to be licensed.

Asterisks indicate states that are in the process of enacting regulations governing recognition of the FPGEC certificate.

Arizona
Arkansas
California
Colorado
Connecticut
Delaware
District of Columbia
Florida
Georgia
Hawaii
Idaho
Illinois
*Indiana
Iowa
Kansas
Kentucky
Maryland
Massachusetts
Michigan
Mississippi
Minnesota
Missouri
Nebraska
Nevada
New Jersey
New Mexico
North Carolina
North Dakota
Ohio
Oklahoma
Oregon
Pennsylvania
Rhode Island
South Carolina
South Dakota
Texas
Vermont
Virginia
Washington
West Virginia

Evaluation of Credentials

Most state boards consider FPGEC certification. A few states, however, may also approve foreign graduates who are not FPGEC certified on the basis of their credentials. For information, contact the appropriate state board.

NABP Resources

NABP offers a variety of publications designed to help pharmacists prepare for licensure. Information on publications that may help you prepare for licensure are listed here. All are available by calling the NABP Publications Desk at (847) 698-6227.

Survey of Pharmacy Law

A comprehensive review of aspects of pharmacy law for the 50 states, the District of Columbia, and Puerto Rico.

Revised annually, the *Survey* consists of four sections: organizational law, licensing law, drug law, and census data. Footnoted charts in each section summarize such areas of concern as the issuance and renewal of licenses, prescribing and dispensing authority, pharmacy technicians, state drug restrictions, and patient counseling requirements. $20.

NAPLEX Computerized Candidate's Review Guide

The purpose of this computerized guide is to help pharmacy students prepare for the NAPLEX. $10.

Other Resources

APhA offers three review books to help students get ready for the NAPLEX and the FDLE: *Comprehensive Pharmacy Review* ($31 for APhA-ASP members), *Comprehensive Pharmacy Review Practice Exams* ($20), and *Strauss's Federal Drug Laws and Examination Review* ($28).

Appendix J

State Boards of Pharmacy

Alabama State Board of Pharmacy
Jerry Moore
Executive Secretary
1 Perimeter Park South
Suite 425 South
Birmingham, AL 35243
205/967-0130

Alaska Board of Pharmacy
Brandi Barger
Licensing Examiner
P.O. Box 110806
Juneau, AK 99811-0806
907/465-2589

Arizona State Board of Pharmacy
L. A. Lloyd
Executive Director
5060 N. 19th Avenue, Suite 101
Phoenix, AZ 85015
602/255-5125

Arkansas State Board of Pharmacy
John T. Douglas
Executive Director
101 E. Capitol, Suite 218
Little Rock, AR 72201
501/682-0190

California State Board of Pharmacy
Patricia F. Harris
Executive Officer
400 R Street, Suite 4070
Sacramento, CA 95814
916/455-5014

Colorado State Board of Pharmacy
Kent Mount
Administrative Officer
1560 Broadway, Suite 1310
Denver, CO 80202-5146
303/894-7750

Connecticut Commission of Pharmacy
Margherita R. Giuliano
Board Administrator
State Office Building
Room G-1A
Hartford, CT 06106
203/566-3290

Delaware State Board of Pharmacy
Bonnie Wallner
Executive Secretary
Jesse Cooper Building
Federal & Water Streets
Dover, DE 19901
302/739-4798

District of Columbia Board of Pharmacy
Cheryl A. Robinson
Secretary
614 H Street, N.W.
Room 904
Washington, DC 20001
202/727-7465

Florida Board of Pharmacy
John D. Taylor
Executive Director
North Wood Center
1940 N. Monroe Street, Suite 60
Tallahassee, FL 32399-0775
904/488-7546

Georgia State Board of Pharmacy
Gregg W. Schuder
Executive Director
State Examining Boards
166 Pryor Street, S.W.
Atlanta, GA 30303
404/656-3912

Hawaii State Board of Pharmacy
Ruth Gushiken
Executive Officer
P.O. Box 3469
Honolulu, HI 96801
808/586-2698

Idaho Board of Pharmacy
Richard "Mick" Markuson
Executive Director
P.O. Box 83720
280 N. 8th Street, Suite 204
Boise, ID 83720-0067
208/334-2356

Illinois Department of Professional Regulation
Nikki M. Zollar
Director
320 W. Washington, 3rd Floor
Springfield, IL 62786
217/785-0800

Appendix J (cont.)

Indiana Board of Pharmacy
Director
Health Professions Bureau
402 W. Washington Street
Room 041
Indianapolis, IN 46204-2739
317/232-1140

Iowa Board of Pharmacy Examiners
Lloyd K. Jessen
Executive Secretary/Director
1209 E. Court
Executive Hills West
Des Moines, IA 50319
515/281-5944

Kansas State Board of Pharmacy
Larry Froelich
Executive Director
Landon State Office Building
900 Jackson, Room 513
Topeka, KS 66612
913/296-4056

Kentucky Board of Pharmacy
Ralph E. Bouvette
Executive Director
1024 Capital Center Drive
Suite 210
Frankfort, KY 40601-8204
502/573-1580

Louisiana Board of Pharmacy
Howard B. Bolton
Executive Director
5615 Corporate Boulevard, Suite 8E
Baton Rouge, LA 70808-2537
504/925-6496

Maine Board of Commissioners of Pharmacy
Alex Severance
Board Coordinator
Department of Professional and Financial Regulation
Division of Licensing and Enforcement
Commission of Pharmacy
State House Station #35
Augusta, ME 04333
207/624-8603

Maryland Board of Pharmacy
Norene Pease
Executive Director
4201 Patterson Avenue
Baltimore, MD 21215-2299
410/764-4755

Massachusetts Board of Registration in Pharmacy
Lori A. Bassinger
Executive Director
100 Cambridge Street, Room 1514
Boston, MA 02202
617/727-9955

Michigan Board of Pharmacy
Carol S. Johnson
Licensing Administrator
Department of Commerce
611 W. Ottawa, 4th Floor
P.O. Box 30018
Lansing, MI 48909
517/373-9102

Minnesota Board of Pharmacy
David E. Holmstrom
Executive Director
2700 University Avenue W., #107
St. Paul, MN 55114-1079
612/642-0541

Mississippi State Board of Pharmacy
William L. "Buck" Stevens
Executive Director
P.O. Box 24507
Jackson, MS 39225-4507
601/354-6750

Missouri Board of Pharmacy
Kevin E. Kinkade
Executive Director
P.O. Box 625
Jefferson City, MO 65102
573/751-0091

Montana Board of Pharmacy
Warren R. Amole, Jr.
Executive Director
510 1st Avenue N., Suite 100
Great Falls, MT 59401
406/761-5131 or 406/444-1698

Nebraska Board of Examiners in Pharmacy
Katherine A. Brown
Executive Secretary
P.O. Box 95007
Lincoln, NE 68509
402/471-2118

Nevada State Board of Pharmacy
Keith W. Macdonald
Executive Secretary
1201 Terminal Way, Suite 212
Reno, NV 89502
702/322-0691

New Hampshire Board of Pharmacy
Paul G. Boisseau
Executive Secretary
57 Regional Drive
Concord, NH 03301-8518
603/271-2350

New Jersey State Board of Pharmacy
H. Lee Gladstein

Executive Director
P.O. Box 45013
Newark, NJ 07101
201/504-6450

New Mexico Board of Pharmacy
Richard W. Thompson
Executive Director
University Towers, Suite 400B
1650 University Boulevard, N.E.
Albuquerque, NM 87102
505/841-9102

New York Board of Pharmacy
Lawrence H. Mokhiber
Executive Secretary
Cultural Education Center
Room 3035
Albany, NY 12230
518/474-3848

North Carolina Board of Pharmacy
David R. Work
Executive Director
P.O. Box 459
Carrboro, NC 27510-0459
919/942-4454

North Dakota State Board of Pharmacy
William J. Grosz
Executive Director
P.O. Box 1354
Bismarck, ND 58502-1354
701/328-9535

Ohio State Board of Pharmacy
Franklin Z. Wickham
Executive Director
77 S. High Street, 17th Floor
Columbus, OH 43266-0320
614/466-4143

Oklahoma State Board of Pharmacy
Bryan H. Potter
Executive Director
4545 Lincoln Boulevard, Suite 112
Oklahoma City, OK 73105-3488
405/521-3815

Oregon State Board of Pharmacy
Ruth A. Vandever
Executive Director
State Office Building, Room 425
800 N.E. Oregon Street, #9
Portland, OR 97232
503/731-4032

Pennsylvania State Board of Pharmacy
W. Richard Marshman
Executive Secretary
124 Pine Street
P.O. Box 2649
Harrisburg, PA 17105-2649
717/783-7157

Puerto Rico Board of Pharmacy
Luisa M. Colom
Executive Director
Department of Health
Office of Regulations and Certification of Health Professionals
Board of Pharmacy
Call Box 10,200
Santurce, PR 00908
809/725-8161

Rhode Island Board of Pharmacy
Norman Phelps
Administrator
Department of Health
Division of Drug Control
3 Capitol Hill, Room 304
Providence, RI 02908-5097
401/277-2837

South Carolina Department of Labor, Licensing, and Regulation Board of Pharmacy
Joseph L. Mullinax II
Executive Director
1026 Sumter Street, Room 209
P.O. Box 11927
Columbia, SC 29211
803/734-1010

South Dakota State Board of Pharmacy
Galen Jordre
Secretary
222 E. Capitol Avenue, Suite 7
P.O. Box 518
Pierre, SD 57501-0518
605/224-2338

Tennessee Board of Pharmacy
Kendall M. Lynch
Director
Volunteer Plaza, Second Floor
500 James Robertson Parkway
Nashville, TN 37243-1149
615/741-2718

Texas State Board of Pharmacy
Fred S. Brinkley, Jr.
Executive Director/Secretary
333 Guadalupe, Tower 3, Suite 600
Austin, TX 78701-3942
512/305-8026

Utah Board of Pharmacy
J. Craig Jackson
Division Director
160 E. 300 South
P.O. Box 45805
Salt Lake City, UT 84145-0805
801/530-6767

Vermont Board of Pharmacy
Carla Preston
Staff Assistant
Office of Professional Regulation

Appendix J (cont.)

109 State Street
Montpelier, VT 05609-1106
802/828-2875

Virginia Board of Pharmacy
Scotti W. Milley
Executive Director
6606 W. Broad Street, Suite 400
Richmond, VA 23230-1717
804/662-9911

Virgin Islands Board of Pharmacy
Nathalie George McDowell
Commissioner of Health
Department of Health
St. Thomas Hospital
48 Sugar Estate
St. Thomas, VI 00802
809/774-0117

Washington State Board of Pharmacy
Donald H. Williams
Executive Director
P.O. Box 47863
Olympia, WA 98504-7863
360/753-6834

West Virginia Board of Pharmacy
Betty Jo Payne
Office Administrator
236 Capitol Street
Charleston, WV 25301
304/558-0558

Wisconsin Pharmacy Examining Board
Patrick D. Braatz
Director, Bureau of Health Professions
1400 E. Washington
P.O. Box 8935
Madison, WI 53708
608/266-0483

Wyoming State Board of Pharmacy
Marilynn H. Mitchell
Executive Director
1720 S. Poplar Street, Suite 5
Casper, WY 82601
307/234-0294

Appendix K

Examination Requirements

State	NABPLEX®/NAPLEX™	FDLE®	State Law	Other	Does State Participate in Score Transfer Program
Alabama	Yes	Yes	Yes	Interview	Yes A
Alaska	Yes	No	Yes I	No	Yes
Arizona	Yes	No	Yes	No	Yes
Arkansas	Yes	No	Yes	No	Yes A
California	No	No	No	Yes J	No
Colorado	Yes	No	Yes	No	Yes
Connecticut	Yes	No	Yes	C,G	Yes
Delaware	Yes	No	Yes	-	Yes A
District of Columbia	Yes	Yes	D.C. Exam	No	Yes A
Florida	Yes	No	Yes	No	B
Georgia	Yes	No	Yes	Yes H	Yes A
Hawaii	Yes	Yes	Yes	-	Yes
Idaho	Yes	No	Yes	No	Yes A
Illinois	Yes	Yes	Yes	No	Yes
Indiana	Yes	Yes	Yes	Yes H	Yes
Iowa	Yes	Yes	Yes	No	Yes
Kansas	Yes	Yes	Yes	-	Yes A
Kentucky	Yes	No	Yes C	Yes C	Yes
Louisiana	Yes	No	Yes	No	Yes A,D,E
Maine	Yes	No	Yes	No	Yes A
Maryland	Yes	No	Yes	Yes E	Yes E
Massachusetts	Yes	No	Yes	No	Yes
Michigan	Yes	No	Yes	No	Yes
Minnesota	Yes	Yes	-	-	Yes A
Mississippi	Yes	No	Yes	No	Yes A
Missouri	Yes	Yes	Yes	No	Yes A
Montana	Yes	No	Yes	-	Yes A
Nebraska	Yes	No	Yes	No	Yes
Nevada	Yes	No	Yes	-	Yes
New Hampshire	Yes	No	Yes	No	Yes
New Jersey	Yes	No	Yes	No	Yes
New Mexico	Yes	No	Yes	No	Yes A
New York	Yes	No	Yes	Yes H	Yes
North Carolina	Yes	No	Yes	Yes	Yes A,E
North Dakota	Yes	Yes	Yes	Yes F	Yes
Ohio	Yes	No	Yes	No	No
Oklahoma	Yes	No	Yes	No	Yes
Oregon	Yes	No	Yes	No	Yes
Pennsylvania	Yes	Yes	No	-	Yes A
Puerto Rico	Yes	No	-	-	-
Rhode Island	Yes	No	Yes	No	Yes
South Carolina	Yes	No	Yes	No	Yes E
South Dakota	Yes	No	Yes	No	Yes
Tennessee	Yes	No	Yes	No	Yes A
Texas	Yes	No	Yes	-	Yes A
Utah	Yes	Yes	Yes	No	Yes A
Vermont	Yes	Yes	Yes	-	Yes
Virginia	Yes	No	Yes I	-	Yes
Washington	Yes	Yes	Yes	No	Yes
West Virginia	Yes	No	Yes	K	No
Wisconsin	Yes	Yes	Yes	Yes	Yes
Wyoming	Yes	Yes	Yes	No	Yes A,E

Laws in all states, including the District of Columbia and Puerto Rico, require applicants for licensure to: (1) have graduated from an accredited first professional degree program of a college of pharmacy; and (2) have passed an examination given by the board of pharmacy. All states, the District of Columbia, and Puerto Rico use the National Association of Boards of Pharmacy Licensure Examination (NABPLEX®)/North American Pharmacist Licensure Examination (NAPLEX™), except California.

Publications concerning the NABPLEX/NAPLEX (Candidate's Review Guide) and Federal Drug Law Examination (FDLE®) are available from the NABP Publications Desk, 700 Busse Highway, Park Ridge, Illinois 60068.

Legend

A – Scores may not be transferred from Florida.

B – Scores may be transferred from Florida to some other state; however, scores may not be transferred to Florida from another state.

C – Jurisprudence; General Pharmacy Practice Examination, including Dispensing Laboratory Examination.

D – Louisiana will score transfer on a reciprocal basis with any other state that will accept Louisiana scores.

E – Applicants licensed by score transfer must wait until the next exam administration to complete remainder of exam requirements (MD—Maryland Law and Maryland Laboratory Exams; SC,WY—law exam).

F – Oral patient consultation examination.

G – Plus pharmaceutical calculations exam.

H – Practical exam.

I – Combined state/federal law exam.

J – California pharmacist licensure examination.

K – Errors and Omissions Exam.

Reprinted with permission from the 1996-97 National Association of Boards of Pharmacy *Survey of Pharmacy Law*.

Practical Experience: Internship Hours

Appendix L responds to the following questions:
1. Amount of practical experience required by the board?
2. Total amount of time required after graduation?
3. What academic year does pharmacy internship/externship credit begin with the board (B.S. program/Pharm.D. program)?
4. Amount of college-supervised experience allowed by the board?

State	1.	2.	3.	4.
Alabama	1,500 R	400 R	First professional year	May be obtained through a college-structured or a nonstructured program, all under the supervision of registered preceptor.
Alaska	1,500 R	None	Third professional year	1,500 hours internship required by board.
Arizona	1,500 R	None	First professional year	1,500 hours required by regulation.
Arkansas	2,000	None	After first professional year	Actual hours accepted for internship in conjunction with academic credit, 1,500 hours for Pharm.D. program. Additional internship credit accepted while enrolled in school, but not in class.
California	1,500 S	1,000 R before taking exam	First professional year	Minimum of 900 hours internship time in a pharmacy under a preceptor's supervision; 600 hours granted at board's discretion, which may include 600 hours clinical clerkship.
Colorado	1,800	None	First professional year	Maximum of 40 hours per week; 1,200 hours may be obtained while enrolled in pharmacy school. Up to 720 hours may be obtained via a clinical rotation. Up to 30 percent of the required hours may be obtained with a drug manufacturer or with a school of pharmacy in drug or drug-related research activities.
Connecticut	1,500	None	After completing two years of college and while enrolled in college of pharmacy	1,500 internship hours while enrolled in ACPE-approved college. Maximum of 40 hours per week. Not more than 400 hours can be credited towards nontraditional experience.
Delaware	1,500	None	First professional year	Full credit for college-supervised programs.
District of Columbia	1,500/1,000 R	-	First professional year	1,000 internship hours while enrolled.
Florida	2,080 (varies)	N/A	First professional year	Varies.
Georgia	1,500 R	-	First professional year	480 hours internship in conjunction with academic credit. 480 hours for B.S. program, 700 hours for Pharm.D. program.
Hawaii	1,500 R	None	After successful completion of first professional year	1,500 hours internship required by board.
Idaho	1,500 R	None	First professional year	1,500 hours internship required by board.
Illinois	400 S	None	First professional year	400 hours internship in conjunction with academic credit.
Indiana	1,040	520	Upon enrollment in pharmacy school	520 hours maximum required by board.
Iowa	1,500 R	None	After two years of full-time college enrollment, one semester of which must be within a college of pharmacy	1,000 hours internship in conjunction with academic credit; additional 500 hours required to be nonconcurrent with academic training.
Kansas	1,500 R, S	None	First professional year	1,000 program hours accepted by board.

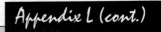

State	1.	2.	3.	4.
Kentucky	1,500	None	After second academic year	Up to 960 hours for Pharm.D. and up to 710 hours for B.S. college programs.
Louisiana	1 year S 1,500 R	500	Final professional year	Minimum of 600 hours before externship; 400 hours in conjunction with academic credit; 1,500 hours total required by board.
Maine	1,500	None	First professional year	1,500 hours required by board.
Maryland	1,560	None	First professional year	Up to 1,560 hours required by board.
Massachusetts	1,500	None	After completion of second year	Internship time while enrolled; 1,500 hours required by board including 400 hours clinical externship.
Michigan	1,000	None	First professional year	40 hours a week while enrolled, but not in classes; 16 hours a week while attending classes; board-approved practical experience within college program varies by college; up to 1,000 hours clinical externship.
Minnesota	1,500	None	After first professional year	400 hours while attending classes; 1,500 hours allowed by board.
Mississippi	1,600	None	First professional year	Up to 800 hours while enrolled but not in classes; 800 hours in conjunction with academic credit.
Missouri	1,500	None	After 30 hours of college of pharmacy credit	750 hours while enrolled but not in classes (externship); 10 hours per week while attending classes, maximum of 500 hours (concurrent); 40 hours per week during summer or academic breaks (nonconcurrent).
Montana	1,500 R	None	After first professional year	700 hours in conjunction with academic credit.
Nebraska	1,500 R	None	After completion of one week of pharmacy school	Up to 640 hours for a B.S. degree and up to 1,300 hours for a Pharm.D. degree in conjunction with academic credit.
Nevada	1,500 S	None	First professional year	500 hours in conjunction with academic credit.
New Hampshire	1,500 R, S	None	Summer preceding first professional year	At discretion of board.
New Jersey	1,000 R	Varies	First professional year	Varies. 1,000 hours required by regulation.
New Mexico	1,500 R	None	After 30 semester hours of college of pharmacy credit	1,000 hours while attending classes; 500 hours in conjunction with academic credit.
New York	6 months R (1,040)	None	After third academic year	Graduates of registered or accredited programs leading to the doctor of pharmacy degree shall be considered to have completed the internship requirement.
North Carolina	1,500	None	After second academic year	Actual hours worked.
North Dakota	1,500	None	Sixth academic year	1,500 hours required by rule.
Ohio	1,500 R	None	After successful completion of 48 semester hours or 72 quarter hours of college and acceptance to a college of pharmacy	Board-approved hours.
Oklahoma	1,500	None	First professional year	Up to 750 hours.
Oregon	2,000	None	First professional and third academic year	Board-approved hours.
Pennsylvania	1,500	None	Third year	Up to 750 hours in conjunction with academic credit.
Puerto Rico	1,500	None	Third year	540 hours in conjunction with academic credit. No more than 40 hours a week internship time while enrolled, but not in classes.
Rhode Island	1,500	None	Third academic year	No more than 40 hours per week. 750 hours in conjunction with academic credit.
South Carolina	1,500 S	None	Three months prior to entering pharmacy school	2 week minimum while enrolled, but not in classes; 500 hours maximum in conjunction with academic credit.

Appendix L (cont.)

State	1.	2.	3.	4.
South Dakota	1,500 R	None	First professional year	1,500 hours allowed; 880 hours must be obtained in settings where training develops general pharmacist competencies.
Tennessee	1,500	None	First professional year	1,100 hours in conjunction with academic credit; 400 hours may be obtained through nontraditional programs.
Texas	1,500 R	None	After completion of 30 credit hours towards a pharmacy degree	1,500 hours allowed by regulation.
Utah	1,500	None	After 15 quarter hours of professional pharmacy courses	900 hours in conjunction with academic credit.
Vermont	1,500 R	None	Third year	Up to 750 hours in conjunction with academic credit.
Virginia	6 months/1,000	None	After first professional year	Up to 6 months and 1,000 hours required by the board.
Washington	1,500	None	After the first quarter/semester of pharmacy education	700 hours in conjunction with academic credit; 1,200 hours for graduates after June 1, 1999.
West Virginia	1,500 S	None	Upon pharmacy school enrollment	500 hours while attending classes; 640 hours allowed by the board.
Wisconsin*	1,500 R	500	Fourth year of pharmacy school curriculum	500 hours allowed by the board.
Wyoming	1,500 R	None	After the first professional year	500 hours of college-supervised clinical clerkship.

* Pharmacy internship under the jurisdiction of the Pharmacy Internship Board, University of Wisconsin, 425 N. Charter Street, Madison, WI 53706.

All jurisdictions require candidates for licensure to have a record of practical experience or internship training acquired under the supervision and instruction of a licensed practitioner.

Legend

R - Required by rule or regulation
S - Required by statute

NABP Internship Committee's definition of "concurrent time" as it applies to internship programs:
We define concurrent time as experience gained while a person is a full-time student. Further, a full-time student is defined as one carrying, in any given school term, at least 75 percent of the average number of credit hours per term needed to graduate within five years.
The 400 concurrent hours may be in any of the three areas or combinations of them: (1) traditional internship supervised by the college, (2) clinical pharmacy programs, and (3) demonstration projects.
In the event that the student is registered in a college-administered practicum which involves the student in a 40-hour work week, he is not to be considered as acquiring concurrent time in this situation. He could be carrying three semester hours or less of didactic, academic work.

Reprinted with permission from the 1996-97 National Association of Boards of Pharmacy *Survey of Pharmacy Law.*

Appendix M

Continuing Pharmaceutical Education Requirements

Forty-nine (49) boards of pharmacy require (or will soon require) that pharmacists participate in continuing-education activities as a prerequisite for relicensure. There are fairly uniform requirements regarding the types of programs that are recognized and the prescribed range of acceptable content matter. Three (3) boards report no activities related to continuing pharmaceutical education.

NOTE: One (1) continuing-education unit, CEU, is equivalent to ten (10) contact hours (1 contact hour = 0.1 CEU).

Boards Requiring Participation in Continuing Pharmaceutical Education for Relicensure

Alabama
By January 1 of each year, every pharmacist must furnish proof of participation in not less than 15 hours of approved continuing education during the preceding year, 3 hours of which must be live exposure. Carry-over of credit is allowed.

Alaska
Each pharmacist seeking renewal of a license shall obtain an average of 15 credit hours of continuing education per year offered by ACPE-approved providers during the previous licensure period. Only programs administered by ACPE-approved providers will be accepted by the board of pharmacy.

Arizona
Pharmacists must satisfactorily complete 3.0 CEUs of continuing professional education activities sponsored by ACPE- or board-approved providers. At least 0.3 CEUs shall be pharmacy law subjects. Satisfactory proof of participation should be retained by participants for five years. No carry-over of credit is allowed.

Arkansas
Requires 30 contact hours (3.0 CEUs) of approved continuing education every two years. Nursing home consultant pharmacists are required to obtain 3 additional hours per year specifically related to consultation.

California
Pharmacists must complete 30 hours of approved continuing pharmaceutical education every two years. All continuing pharmaceutical education providers must be ACPE-approved providers or recognized by the Accreditation Evaluation Service (AES). Providers who are not ACPE- or AES-approved may petition the board for approval of courses. Pharmacists may independently petition as well. No carry-over of credit is allowed.

Connecticut
Pharmacists are required to complete 15 hours of continuing education in the previous calendar year (January to December). At least 5 of those hours MUST be at a live presentation. Only courses that are ACPE-, CME-, CNE-, or commission-approved are accepted.

Delaware
Pharmacists must obtain 30 hours of continuing pharmaceutical education during each biennial renewal period. No carry-over of credit is allowed.

Florida
Biennial renewal certificates require satisfactory proof that during the two years prior to the renewal application the licensee has participated in not less than 15 hours PER CALENDAR YEAR of approved continuing professional education programs. In addition, 12 hours of consultant pharmacist course work is required annually for biennial renewal of a consultant license. Additionally, 24 hours of nuclear pharmacist course work is required for biennial renewal of a nuclear license. A board-approved 3-hour course on AIDS/HIV is required prior to licensure and renewal of licensure.

Georgia
Pharmacists must obtain 30 hours (3.0 CEUs) of continuing pharmaceutical education credit every two years as a condition of relicensure. All ACPE-approved providers giving a program in Georgia are required to submit a copy of the Program Description Form to the Georgia State Board of Pharmacy 60 days prior to the date of the program. Non-ACPE-approved providers must apply for and obtain a Georgia Board of Pharmacy I.D. number for each program and have a 60-day prior approval for their programs.

Idaho
134. Amount of Continuing Education. The equivalent of one and one-half (1.5) continuing-education units (CEU) shall be required annually of each applicant for renewal of license. One continuing-education unit is the equivalent of ten (10) clock hours of participation in programs approved by the Board of Pharmacy.
(07-01-93)

01. ACPE, CME. At a minimum, eight clock hours (0.8 CEU) will be all or a combination of American Council on Pharmaceutical Education (ACPE) or Continuing Medical Education (CME) approved programs. (12-7-94)

02. Pharmacy law. One clock hour (0.1 CEU) must be board of pharmacy-approved jurisprudence (pharmacy law) programs.
(07-01-93)

03. Non-ACPE. A maximum of six clock hours (0.6 CEU) may be non-ACPE approved programs. (12-7-94)

Illinois
Pharmacists must obtain 30 hours (3.0 CEUs) of pharmacy continuing education from ACPE-approved providers during the two calendar years preceding expiration of certificate.

Indiana
Pharmacists are required to complete 30 hours of approved continuing education every two years. No more than six hours of business- or computer-related CE is accepted. No carry-over of credit is allowed. At least half of total hours must be ACPE-approved.

Iowa
Requires 30 hours (3.0 CEUs) of approved continuing pharmaceutical education every two years as a condition for license renewal. No carry-over of credit is allowed. Fifty percent of CE must be in drug therapy-related course work from an ACPE-approved provider.

Kansas
Requires 15 hours (1.5 CEUs) of approved continuing pharmaceutical education for annual registration. No carry-over of credit is allowed.

Kentucky
Each licensee is required to complete a minimum of 15 hours (1.5 CEUs) annually in accredited programs. One hour per year must be from a Kentucky Cabinet for Human Resources-approved HIV/AIDS program. Non-ACPE-approved programs must contain the Kentucky Board of Pharmacy I.D. number. Non-ACPE-approved courses given out of state are not reviewed for credit. Credit must be obtained between January 1 and December 31 each year. No carry-over credit is permitted.

Appendix M (cont.)

Louisiana
Fifteen (15) hours (1.5 CEUs) of continuing pharmaceutical education from ACPE-approved providers must be completed annually as a prerequisite for relicensure. No carry-over of credit is allowed.

Maine
Pharmacists must submit satisfactory proof of participation in not less than 15 hours of approved programs of continuing pharmaceutical education during the preceding calendar year. No carry-over of credit is allowed.

Maryland
To qualify for biennial license renewal, pharmacists must have accumulated 30 hours of continuing-education credit in approved programs. No carry-over of credit is allowed.

Massachusetts
Pharmacists must complete 15 hours (1.5 CEUs) of continuing pharmaceutical education every year (30 hours [3.0 CEUs] per two-year renewal period). No carry-over of credit is allowed from year to year. Of the 15 hours required per year, at least 2 hours shall be in the area of pharmacy law; at least 5 hours shall be from live programs; and not more than 10 hours shall be credited through correspondence courses.

Michigan
To qualify for biennial license renewal, pharmacists must have accumulated 30 hours of continuing-education credit in approved programs. No carry-over of credit is allowed.

Minnesota
Requires at least 30 hours of credit from accredited continuing-education programs every two years. Carry-over and splitting of program hours are not allowed.

Mississippi
Pharmacists are required to submit to the Board of Pharmacy evidence of completion of 20 hours (2.0 CEUs) in approved programs every two years. No carry-over of credit is allowed. Six hours must be obtained by contact participation.

Missouri
Pharmacists are required to submit proof of 10 hours (1.0 CEUs) of continuing pharmaceutical education for annual license renewal. No carry-over of credit is allowed.

Montana
Pharmacists are required to participate in 15 hours (1.5 CEUs) of approved programs each year following the first license renewal. A minimum of 5 hours (0.5 CEUs) is to be obtained in approved group (i.e., live) programs. One-year carry-over of credit is allowed.

Nebraska
Every two years, pharmacists will be required to complete 30 hours of continuing pharmaceutical education sponsored by ACPE-approved providers. Each pharmacist is responsible for keeping his or her own records.

Nevada
Pharmacists must submit proof of receiving 30 hours of continuing-education credit within the two years preceding the current renewal period. In-state registrants must have 15 hours in accredited programs, including one hour in a jurisprudence program. Out-of-state registrants may submit 30 hours of acceptable continuing education. Carry-over of credits is not allowed.

New Hampshire
Requires 15 hours (1.5 CEUs) for annual relicensure. A minimum of 5 hours (0.5 CEUs) must be didactic (live presentation) hours. No carry-over of credit is allowed. Programs must be from ACPE-approved providers or approved by any board of pharmacy or AMA Category I accredited.

New Jersey
Effective April 11, 1995, legislation was enacted that transfers authority for continuing pharmaceutical education to the Board of Pharmacy.
Chapter 79, C.45:14-11.11. Continuing education required of pharmacists. 1. The Board of Pharmacy of the State of New Jersey shall require each person registered as a pharmacist, as a condition for biennial certification pursuant to R.S. 45:14-11 and P.L. 1972, c. 108 (C.45:1-7), to complete 30 credits of continuing pharmaceutical education and submit proof thereof, as provided in section 2 of this act, during each biennial registration period. C.45:14-11.12. Standards for continuing education. 2. a. The Board shall: (1) Establish standards for continuing pharmaceutical education, including the subject matter and content of courses of study, the selection of instructors, and the type of continuing-education credits required of a registered pharmacist as a condition for biennial certification; (2) Approve educational programs offering credit towards the continuing pharmaceutical education requirements; and (3) Approve other equivalent educational programs, including, but not limited to, home study courses, and shall establish procedures for the issuance of credit upon satisfactory proof of the completion of these programs. b. In the case of education courses and programs, each hour of instruction shall be equivalent to one credit.

Effective May 1, 1995, the board voted to automatically accept ACPE-approved continuing-education credits. Programs presented by non-ACPE providers must apply to the board for approval of these presentations for accreditation. There is a $50 fee for this review. Individuals attending non-ACPE programs who wish to receive continuing-education credit can have these programs reviewed for a $10 fee. Non-ACPE courses must be issued a New Jersey number to be acceptable for continuing-education credit.

New Mexico
Pharmacists are required to submit evidence of 15 hours (1.5 CEUs) of continuing pharmaceutical education offered by ACPE-approved providers to renew their annual registration. A maximum of 15 hours, or one year of credit, may be accrued in excess and carried over to the next licensure year. One hour must be in the area of pharmacy law. Resident pharmacists must attend a program presented by the inspection staff. Nonresident pharmacists may take an ACPE-accredited law course.

New York
During each triennial registration period, pharmacists must complete a minimum of 45 hours of acceptable formal continuing education with no more than 22 hours consisting of self-study courses.

North Carolina
Requires 10 hours (1.0 CEUs) of continuing pharmaceutical education per year, with no more than 5 hours (0.5 CEUs) of noncontact (i.e., correspondence/home-study) program credit.

North Dakota
Requires 30 hours (3.0 CEUs) of continuing pharmaceutical education offered by ACPE-approved providers every two years for license renewal. One-year carry-over of credit is allowed.

Ohio
Requires that evidence of 4.5 CEUs of continuing pharmaceutical education offered by approved providers be submitted at intervals of three years. 0.3 CEUs must be in board-approved jurisprudence courses. No carry-over of credit is allowed.

Oklahoma
Relicensure or licensure by reciprocity requires satisfactory proof of not less than 15 clock hours of participation in accredited continuing-education programs per year. Carry-over of credit is not allowed.

Oregon
Each year pharmacists must satisfactorily complete 15 hours (1.5 CEUs) in approved continuing-education programs OR must pass a continuing-education examination given by the board no later than eight months prior to the next date for renewal of the annual license. If applicant passes the open book examination with a score of not less than 90 percent, the board will certify the applicant as having met the continuing pharmacy education requirement for license renewal. One hour of credit will not be allowed for taking the examination. Eleven of the 15 hours must be in law and/or therapeutics; one hour must be in law; four hours may be in socioeconomic areas. No carry-over of credit is allowed.

Pennsylvania
Pharmacists are required to complete a minimum of 30 credit hours (3.0 CEUs) of continuing education offered by ACPE-approved providers every two years. No carry-over of credit is allowed.

Appendix M (cont.)

Puerto Rico

Pharmacists must complete 35 hours (3.5 CEUs) of continuing pharmaceutical education for recertification every three years, with a minimum of 10 hours per year. The only acceptable programs are those offered by ACPE or providers approved by the Puerto Rico Board of Pharmacy.

Rhode Island

Pharmacists must complete 15 hours (1.5 CEUs) of continuing education offered by approved providers. Five (5) hours of credit must be obtained through participation in live programs. No carry-over of credit is allowed.

South Carolina

Pharmacists must complete 15 hours of approved continuing education to be eligible for active license renewal. At least 6 hours of the total must be from live presentations. At least 7.5 hours must be concerning drug therapy or patient management. Excess credits may be carried forward one calendar year.

South Dakota

Pharmacists must provide evidence of completion of 12 hours of continuing education in approved programs in order to be eligible for annual relicensure.

Tennessee

Pharmacists must complete 30 hours of continuing pharmaceutical education every two years for license renewal. No carry-over of credit is allowed.

Texas

Pharmacists must complete 12 hours of approved CE each year in order to renew their licenses. Up to 12 hours may be carried over to the next license year when excess hours are earned.

Utah

Pharmacists shall complete 24 hours of continuing professional education approved by the division and the Board every two calendar years, beginning January 1, 1993. A minimum of 8 hours must be obtained through attendance at approved lectures, seminars, or workshops and a minimum of 6 hours must be in drug therapy or patient management. Continuing-education hours for licensees who have not been licensed for the entire year will be prorated from the date of licensure at a rate of one hour for each month of licensure. No continuing-education hours may be accrued as excess and carried forward to the succeeding reporting period. Postgraduate studies in an accredited college of pharmacy shall be considered as continuing-education activities. An approved provider is an individual, institution, organization, association, corporation, or agency that has been approved by the American Council on Pharmaceutical Education (ACPE) and regional meetings sponsored by the Utah Pharmaceutical Association.

Vermont

The licensee must complete at least 15 hours (1.5 CEUs), of which at least 0.5 CEUs shall be obtained during participation in a didactic session, for each full year since the date that the applicant's latest license was issued; for a total of 3.0 CEUs per renewal period.

Virginia

§54.1-3314.1 Continuing-education requirements; exemptions; extensions; procedures; out-of-state licensees; nonpractice licenses. A. Each pharmacist shall have obtained a minimum of 15 continuing-education hours of pharmaceutical education through an approved continuing pharmaceutical education program during the year immediately preceding his license renewal date. B. An approved continuing pharmaceutical education program shall be any program approved by the Board. C. Pharmacists who have been initially licensed by the Board during the one year preceding the license renewal date shall not be required to comply with the requirement on the first license renewal date that would immediately follow. D. The Board may grant an exemption from the continuing-education requirement if the pharmacist presents evidence that failure to comply was due to circumstances beyond the control of the pharmacist. E. Upon the written request of a pharmacist, the Board may grant an extension of one year in order for a pharmacist to fulfill the continuing-education requirements for the period of time in question. Such extension shall not relieve the pharmacist of complying with the continuing-education requirement for the current period. F. The pharmacist shall attest to the fact that he has completed the continuing-education requirements as specified by the Board. G. The following shall apply to the requirements for continuing pharmaceutical education: 1. The provider of an approved continuing-education program shall issue to each pharmacist who has successfully completed a program certification that the pharmacist has completed a specified number of hours. 2. The certificates so issued to the pharmacist shall be maintained by the pharmacist for a period of two years following the renewal of his license. 3. The pharmacist shall provide the Board, upon request, with certification of completion of continuing-education programs in a manner to be determined by the Board. H. Pharmacists who are also licensed in other states and who have obtained a minimum of 15 hours of approved continuing-education requirements of such other states need not obtain additional hours. I. The Board shall provide for an inactive status for those pharmacists who do not wish to practice in Virginia. The Board shall require upon request for change from inactive to active status proof of continuing-education hours equal to that which would have been required should the pharmacist have continued to hold an active license. No person shall practice in Virginia unless he holds a current active license.

Washington

Pharmacists are required to complete 15 hours (1.5 CEUs) of professional continuing education as a prerequisite for annual license renewal. No carry-over of credit is allowed.

West Virginia

Fifteen hours (1.5 CEUs) required during previous year to renew license.

Wyoming

Each pharmacist must complete a minimum of 6 credit hours (0.6 CEUs) of accredited continuing pharmaceutical education each year. Carry-over of credit is allowed for one year. Those who have been inactive must demonstrate completion of back-CE for a maximum of five years prior to reactivation.

Boards of Pharmacy that Have Been Granted Legislative Authority to Promulgate Regulations:

District of Columbia

Enabling legislation was passed by the city council, and the board of pharmacy published requirements for 1.5 CEUs for the 1991 renewal period to expand to 3.0 CEUs per renewal period.

States Reporting No Related Activities:

Colorado, Hawaii, and Wisconsin

For additional information regarding specific requirements, please contact the appropriate board of pharmacy.

For additional copies of this report or information about the ACPE Provider Approval Program, please contact American Council on Pharmaceutical Education, Division of Continuing Education, 311 W. Superior Street, Suite 512, Chicago, Illinois 60610; 312/664-3575.

Reprinted with permission from the 1996-97 National Association of Boards of Pharmacy *Survey of Pharmacy Law*.

Licensure Transfer Requirements

State	Fee for Transfer of Licensure	Special Conditions/ Requirements	State Jurisprudence Exam Required?	State	Fee for Transfer of Licensure	Special Conditions/ Requirements	State Jurisprudence Exam Required?
Alabama	$300	A	Yes	New Jersey	$125	A,B,C,F	Yes
Alaska	$230	A	Yes	New Mexico	$200	C	Yes
Arizona	$300	B	Yes	New York	$270 N	F	Yes
Arkansas	$200	F	Yes	North Carolina	$300	F	Yes
California	—	—	—	North Dakota	$150	E	Yes
Colorado	$219	F	Yes	Ohio	$225	J	No
Connecticut	$100	A,D,F	Yes	Oklahoma	$200	B	Yes
Delaware	$150	B	Yes	Oregon	$200 P	E	Yes
District of Columbia	$ 80	T	D.C. law exam	Pennsylvania	$100 Q	A	No
Florida	—	—	—	Puerto Rico	$100	E	Yes
Georgia	$300	F	—	Rhode Island	$100	A,C	Yes
Hawaii	$ 15 I	A,B,C,G	Yes	South Carolina	$350 P	C	Yes
Idaho	$250	A	Yes	South Dakota	$150	E	Yes
Illinois	$200	C,H	No	Tennessee	$300	E	Yes
Indiana	$ 40	B	Yes	Texas	$250 P	A,C,R,S	Yes
Iowa	$150	—	Yes (monthly)	Utah	$100	T	Yes
Kansas	$250	E	Yes	Vermont	$130 N	-	Yes
Kentucky	$250	A,C,F,J	Yes	Virginia	$ 50 U	-	Yes
Louisiana	$150	F	Yes	Washington	$250	A	Yes (monthly)
Maine	$150	K	Yes	West Virginia	$255	V	Yes
Maryland	$200	B	No L	Wisconsin	$250	A,B	Yes
Massachusetts	$100	A	Yes	Wyoming	$200	Interview G	Yes
Michigan	$165	—	Yes				
Minnesota	$175	A,F	Yes (written and oral)				
Mississippi	$200	K	Yes				
Missouri	$350	F,M	Yes				
Montana	$250	—	Yes				
Nebraska	$251	F	Yes				
Nevada	$250 N	A,C	Yes				
New Hampshire	$200	A,C,O	Yes				

The basic rule for pharmaceutic licensure transfer: An applicant must have had the legal qualifications at the time of examination and registration in the state from which he or she applies, which would at that time have enabled him or her to qualify for examination and registration in the state to which he or she applies for licensure transfer registration.

Almost all jurisdictions that grant licensure by licensure transfer (all except California and Florida) require that a pharmacist who applies for such licensure furnish evidence of having acquired a license by examination in a state that grants licensure by licensure transfer. It is necessary that this license be in good standing, as the license by examination is the basis for transferring the license to other licensure transfer states.

Appendix N (cont.)

LEGEND

A – Photographs, identification, and special forms furnished by state in addition to official NABP application. (HI - no photograph required.)

B – There may be restrictions or special requirements for those licensed pharmacists who have not been actively practicing or for those who have been licensed for less than one year. Contact the state board of pharmacy office for details.

C – Licensure transfer applicant must have graduated and received a baccalaureate in pharmacy or a Pharm.D. from a college of pharmacy whose degree program is accredited by ACPE and approved by the board (KY, NV, NM, RI, SC, TX - or applicant must show proof of full FPGEC Certification; KY - FPGEC Certification must have been obtained after October 1992).

D – Examination in math.

E – "F" legend item (below) applicable only to licensees from those states that impose such a preclusion on licensure transfer applicants.

F – Pharmacists who have not been licensed one year are not eligible to be licensed by licensure transfer (AR - six months; KY - Applicants for licensure transfer have the option to sit for the KY portion of the licensure exam and successfully pass the exam which is given twice a year and which includes a wet lab; NY - pharmacists who have not practiced for one year).

G – State of original licensure must have similar licensing requirements.

H – Orientation session required.

I – $15 application fee plus $150 NABPLEX, $30 FDLE, or $60 state jurisprudence exam fees, if applicable.

J – Standards at discretion of the board.

K – Examination discretionary - usually none other than oral.

L – No exam, but written Maryland Law Review required.

M – "E" may be waived if internship is comparable to internship requirements of state.

N – Includes fees for application and initial license where such fees are applicable.

O – Licensure transfer applicant originally licensed after July 1, 1978, must show proof of having passed NABPLEX/NAPLEX.

P – Additional license fee.

Q – Application fee is $25. FDLE required only of persons licensed after April 1, 1983; fee is $75.

R – Applicant's state of initial licensure must grant reciprocal licensure to pharmacists licensed by examination in this state.

S – Licensure transfer applicant originally licensed after January 1, 1978, must show proof of having passed NABPLEX/NAPLEX or equivalent examination based on criteria no less stringent than the criteria in force in this state or demonstrate licensure in good standing for a period of two years immediately prior to the application for licensure transfer.

T – Plus FDLE (UT - if documents at least 2,000 hours of pharmacy practice, FDLE is waived).

U – Plus $125 for law exam.

V – Errors and Omissions Exam.

Reprinted with permission from the 1996-97 National Association of Boards of Pharmacy *Survey of Pharmacy Law*.

Chapter 8

Landing Your First Position

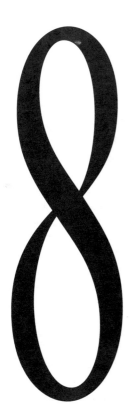

Introduction

When you entered pharmacy school, you took the first step toward your career. Soon you were confronted with a second decision: Which career within the pharmacy profession should you choose?

As you know by now, the opportunities are wide ranging. Pharmacists work in any setting where medications are used. They work with physicians and nurses, to be sure. They also work with veterinarians and dentists. Pharmacists work in independent and chain pharmacies, hospitals, clinics, managed care organizations, nursing homes, poison control centers, and home health care organizations. Pharmacists who work in health systems may be specialists or generalists. Finally, they may focus on pharmacy practice or management.

Pharmacists also teach at colleges and universities. They work in the pharmaceutical and chemical industries. They work for government agencies such as the Public Health Service, Food and Drug Administration, and National Institutes of Health. They find employment in the U.S. armed forces. Pharmacists with management skills have rewarding careers in national and state pharmacy associations. There are pharmacist-lawyers as well as pharmacists who specialize in the development and application of information technology.

This chapter provides some practical advice on how to find the pharmacy career that's best for you. It includes information on résumé writing, interviewing, and other skills that you'll need now and throughout your career.

Job versus Career: What's the Difference?

What's the difference between a job and a career? Here's what Webster's Ninth New Collegiate Dictionary has to say.
• A job is "something that has to be done" or "a specific duty, role or function" or "a regular remunerative position."
• A career is "a profession for which one trains and which is undertaken as a permanent calling."

Which are you looking for? Once you've devoted five or six years of education to the study of pharmacy, the answer is clear. You're looking for a career. Your search may take time and effort. Ultimately, it will be worth it.

Never consider a position that is "just a job." You have too much invested to languish in this type of work.

Taking the First Steps in Your Career

Where do you want to begin? Only you can decide what career path is right for you.

As you prepare to make that decision, it's important to be aware of your options. Equally important is to realize that hardly anyone stays in the same position, from licensure through retirement, anymore. Times change, health care changes, people change, and the profession changes.

Think about the career profiles in Chapter 1. All the interviewees had worked in a number of settings. In so doing, they had acquired new skills and polished old ones. Many worked for a few years before going back to school to earn a Pharm.D. or an M.B.A. degree or to complete a residency or fellowship. Much of their know-how was acquired in the workplace. Many of them took a chance by carving out a role for themselves in a new area such as computer technology. At midcareer or later, they were still growing. The moral of the story is clear: If you make a career choice that doesn't meet your expectations, learn from it and move on.

Stay open-minded. Have fun, take challenges, and don't be afraid to follow your dream. Every career has advantages and disadvantages. What counts is finding the one that suits you best.

Lay the Groundwork

Your career search will take some planning and research. A good starting point is the people right around you. Inquire about the background and experience of your boss, a favorite professor, or mentor.

Ask people in the field you're interested in what they like best about their careers. Walk into a pharmacy, introduce yourself, and set up a date to talk to one or two of the pharmacists about their career paths.

Or perhaps you want to apply your pharmacy knowledge in a totally different arena. Suppose, for example, that you've always been interested in health care policy and want to be a legislative assistant to a lawmaker who works with health issues. Find out who chairs a congressional committee that deals with health matters and write to his or her office, asking how to get involved in that area. Don't just ask how to get a job; ask about training and special skills you would need to have a career in the legislative arena.

You may want to take a few courses in business or marketing. Another important step is to get involved in professional organizations such as the APhA Academy of Students of Pharmacy and pharmacy fraternities. Membership will bring you into contact with pharmacists in different practice settings. You can meet them at alumni functions; at continuing-education programs; at local, state, regional, and national pharmacy association meetings; during an internship or residency; through professors and their contacts; or even while being interviewed for a position.

Consult print resources as well. One excellent reference is *The Pfizer Guide: Pharmacy Career Opportunities*, which covers virtually every type of pharmacist practice.

Find Out Who You Are

To realize your career goals, you must know yourself. This requires a self-assessment.

If you're in your early twenties, your life is probably still in flux. Nonetheless, begin where you are, not where you (or a parent, teacher, or colleague) think you should be. In what areas of pharmacy school did you excel? Where did you feel most comfortable? Where were you less confident? Base your plans on who you are today and the areas of pharmacy that really excite you.

You might find it helpful to visit the career center at your college. Staff may be able to answer some of your general questions. They may also administer psychological assessment tests at your request.

Another assessment technique is to consult close friends, employers, mentors, or other people who have known you for a few years. Ask them for a candid assessment of your strengths and weaknesses. Be sure that they consider your temperament as well as your intellectual capability. Reassure your evaluators that it's okay to offer constructive criticism. It's helpful if they let you know, for instance, that you have a "short fuse" in dealing with others. This feedback might indicate that you would perform better in a career where you are not in constant contact with others, such as research, rather than community pharmacy.

Six Key Questions

Richard Bolles, author of the classic job-hunter's manual *What Color Is Your Parachute?*, outlines six questions for researching who you are and identifying your ideal career.

1. What skills do you have and enjoy using?
2. Where do you want to use these skills?
3. What kinds of organizations can you focus on (in terms of goals and use of your skills) in your geographical area of preference?
4. What are the names of these organizations?
5. What are the problems at the level at which you want to work?
6. Who has the power to hire you?

Fine-Tune Your Search

As you begin to narrow your career search, continue to ask questions. Salary is one of the most important, especially if you have student loans to repay and family responsibilities. But don't get hung up on it. Never make a decision on the basis of salary alone. Remember the words of John Parisi, one of the pharmacists interviewed in Chapter 1: "Don't sell out for a few thousand dollars. Don't take a job that you really hate just because you are going to get paid a few thousand dollars more. Find the practice you want, and the rewards will come."

Far more important than a few thousand dollars' difference in an initial starting salary is developing money-management skills early in life that will enable you to build a sound financial future.

In addition, find out about

the following:
- Opportunity for advancement
- Relocation expenses (if applicable)
- Vacation, sick leave, holidays, personal leave
- Bonuses (for holidays, outstanding individual performance, company performance)
- Reimbursement for continuing education or pursuit of advanced training
- Medical, dental, and life insurance
- Short- and long-term disability insurance
- Retirement plans
- Company car
- Stock options
- Parking or transportation allowance
- Policies on family leave and child care
- Reimbursement for membership in professional associations
- Opportunities for professional travel
- Other benefits (e.g., membership in a fitness center, discounts)

If you expect to be in a position for a short period of time, your priorities will be different than if you are considering long-term employment. Immediate benefits such as salary and leave time will be more important than opportunities for advancement and the company's retirement plan.

Sources of Career Information

Career information is available from a variety of sources. The most common are listed here.

Pharmacy Schools

Your school of pharmacy is a prime place to look for contacts and career ideas. Although most schools do not have a formal career placement center, they do help their students find employment in many ways.

Career Days. Nearly all schools of pharmacy host career days once or twice a year. During these events, representatives of companies that hire pharmacists visit the campus to interview applicants. Organizations that send representatives to these events include chain pharmacies, pharmaceutical companies, the U.S. armed forces, academic health centers, and large independent pharmacies.

You may have to register in advance to participate in the career day interviews. Once you've made an appointment, you will probably be asked to submit a résumé in advance.

Contact your school's career office or the dean's office for more information.

Faculty Members. If you know what area or specialty you'd like to pursue, talk with professors in that area. They are often aware of vacancies and know to whom inquiries should be addressed.

At least one school of pharmacy has designated an informal "career placement professor" who coordinates the school's clerkship program. Because this professor knows most of the area practitioners as well as the students, he's well qualified to act as a "matchmaker." Practitioners routinely call him when they have openings. Students can find summer or temporary work through him as well. Your school may have similar professors. Ask around.

Alumni Relations Offices. A few alumni relations offices have career placement centers. If your school has one, be sure to take advantage of it.

Professional Placement Services

Professional placement services (also known as employment agencies) try to match a person's skills with those that an employer requires for a specific position. Many of these services charge a fee; this may be paid by the employer or the applicant. These services are generally more valuable for mid- or upper-level positions than for entry-level positions; however, they can help you gather information about prospective employers.

On-Line Information

The Internet has a number of employment listings, several of which are listed at the end of this chapter. Some postings are for specific practice areas such as institutional practice and some are combination listings. Look at as many as you can.

State Pharmacy Associations, Societies, and Boards of Pharmacy

Membership in your state pharmacy association or society offers you access to many resources, including pharmacists who know what the working world is like and where positions are available. APhA Midyear Regional and Annual Meetings give you the opportunity to meet pharmacists from beyond your state.

Most state pharmacy associations do not offer formal career placement services. One state association does publish the names and telephone numbers of first- and fifth-year pharmacy students in its newsletter every year to help students get summer jobs. Employers often call their state association to announce openings and ask for referrals. If you're looking, make sure the staff at your state association know your name and telephone number!

Some state associations offer career days similar to those offered by pharmacy schools. These events may be held in conjunction with an annual meeting, as a separate function, or in conjunction with a school of pharmacy. Call your state association for more information. Be sure to ask if the interviewers will be recruiting for entry-level positions.

Classified Advertisements

State and national association pharmacy journals such as the *Journal of the American Pharmaceutical Association* list employment opportunities in their classified advertisement sections.

Ads in newspapers may also be helpful, especially in urban areas.

Many people use these ads successfully. At best, however, they should be considered a supplement to your career search.

Networking

What is networking and how does it fit into your career search? Networking is simply maintaining relationships with people. To be an effective networker, you should never "burn bridges" when you move to a new phase of life. You may find you want to cross the same river twice!

Some people believe they should network only with people with greater experience or influence than they. In truth, the best network links are people like you—people who are interested in similar practices but who may be at a different level or with a different employer. Think of your network as an expanding group of friends who are genuinely interested in helping each other. If you use networking in this way, you will not only get a lot of satisfaction out of your relationships but also find support when you need it.

Once you've made the commitment, networking is easy. For example, suppose you're attending an APhA Midyear Regional Meeting and you come upon a speaker, company representative, or practitioner who has a position similar to one in which you are interested. Walk over and introduce yourself. Many of these people are at the meeting because they want to meet students. They're just as interested in you as you are in them!

Fraternities, sororities, honor societies, and other organizations provide a rich source of networking possibilities. If you're not already a member, consider joining one. Membership can open doors for you not only while you're still in school but throughout your career. You never know when you are going to meet someone who is affiliated with your group. This bond creates an immediate avenue for conversation and sharing of information. Letting this group of friends know that you are looking for a position will instantly expand your career search.

This principle applies equally well to involvement in community and civic organizations—everything from leading a Boy Scout or Girl Scout troop to being a member of a local Kiwanis Club, Toastmasters, or religious organization.

Make sure that people you have met during summer jobs, internships, and residencies remain in your network. Former supervisors are especially important.

In summary, cover your bases. When you're looking for a position, tell everyone. If you introduce yourself to a person and discover that he or she doesn't have anything to offer right now, don't close the door! Stay in touch. Things change, and future career paths are impossible to predict.

Applying for a Position: Cover Letters, Résumés, and Curricula Vitae

Your résumé or curriculum vitae is your calling card. The accompanying cover letter is your chance to introduce yourself. Both should be prepared with meticulous attention to detail.

Cover Letters

Tailor your cover letter to the position for which you are applying. Highlight your qualifications and emphasize how they meet the position description. A sample cover letter is found in Appendix O.

Résumés and Vitas

The difference between a résumé and a curriculum vitae (often called a vita) is the degree of detail that each provides.

- A vita is an exhaustive list of everything that you've done professionally, including research projects, proposals written and grants received, other funding or awards, lectures or other professional talks, publications (including articles, abstracts, and book chapters), and any other professional endeavor in which you've been involved. A vita is essential for a career in academia or research.
- A résumé is usually no more than two pages long. It highlights your educational and professional experience and accomplishments, including awards and honors. Appendix P is a sample résumé; Appendix Q is a sample curriculum vitae.

If you are applying for an academic position, you should probably submit a vita. This is especially true if you are applying for a tenure-track position that entails research. Most other employers will be satisfied with a résumé. Don't send a vita if only a résumé is needed; the interviewer may skip it because of its daunting length!

If the position announcement does not specify, come prepared. Bring both a résumé and a vita.

Do's and Don't's for Résumé and Vita Writers

Many employers use résumés and cover letters as screening tools. A sloppy, poorly written letter will end up at the bottom of the pile or in the waste bin. Spend the time to make your résumé reflect the quality person that you are and the unique talents that you will bring to your future employer.

Decide how you want to organize your résumé. There are two major choices: chronological or functional. The chronological style lists your positions in order of occurrence, starting with the most recent and working backward. The functional style is organized by skills. It combines similar skills that have been acquired in different positions. Draft your résumé both ways and choose the one you like best.

Do's

- Be sure your résumé is visually appealing, clean, and well organized. Have a friend check it for misspellings, grammatical mistakes, and inconsistencies.
- Employers spend an average of 45 seconds looking at each résumé during the initial screening. For this reason, your résumé must yield pertinent information quickly. Use subheads (e.g., Education, Professional Experience) to indicate what information follows.
- As a student you don't have a lot of work experience. For this reason, it's best to list your educational accomplishments first. Your employer is purchasing your education, not your experience.
- Keep your résumé to less than two pages unless the position requires more.
- Get the most out of your words: use "action" words (e.g., created, coordinated, directed, developed, organized) to describe your previous duties.
- Describe the results of your work in quantifiable terms if possible.
- Cut out unnecessary words and examples. If you've done a similar task in more than one position, describe it in detail only one time.
- Keep your résumé on a computer disk or hard drive and update it frequently.

Don'ts

- Don't be egotistical. There's a fine line between promoting yourself and sounding overaggressive. Avoid exaggerated generalizations, such as, "My chapter's membership grew 75% in one year because of me." (Did you personally recruit each member?) Such claims may hurt your credibility.
- Don't include a career objective on your résumé unless it is specifically related to the position for which you are applying. Although you may feel certain that the position matches your career objective perfectly, this may not be equally clear to your interviewer. Do, however, have a career objective in mind and be prepared to discuss it.
- Don't include references. Simply note "References available upon request" at the bottom of the last page of your résumé and have a typed list of names and addresses ready in case the employer requests it. Some suggest leaving this phrase off entirely because employers often routinely request letters of reference with an application for employment.
- Don't include personal information such as marital status, family information, or hobbies.
- Don't title your résumé "Résumé"; this is redundant.

The Employment Interview

Your résumé got you in the door; now your job is to present yourself as a competent professional. What's important at this stage of your career search?

Advance Work

Prepare yourself. Find out as much as you can about your potential employer and the position for which you have applied. Ask for informational materials to be sent to you well before the interview. Read them carefully. Jot down some questions.

The better prepared you are, the more confident you will be, and confidence is essential.

During the Interview

Listen to each question. Make sure that you hear all of it before you begin answering. If it is a multiple-part question, ask the interviewer to repeat each section if necessary.

Answer each question in two minutes or less. If you don't restrict your time, you may begin rambling. The interviewer may want to ask you several questions in a limited amount of time. The less time you talk (while still adequately describing your qualifications), the more time for the interviewer to give you information about the position. You can use this information to your advantage during the rest of the interview.

Remember that you don't have to answer all questions. Interviewers are legally not allowed to ask about marital status, religion, disability history, or other personal information. If you volunteer this type of information, however, it is open for discussion.

Do everything you can to convince a prospective employer that you have the needed skills and qualifications, but never exaggerate to fit the employer's requirements. Doing so would only be cheating yourself. It would force you to conform to what the employer wants you to be rather than to find a position that conforms to what you want.

Interview Etiquette

Look good, look neat, look professional. You don't need to buy new clothes; the interviewer knows you are a student with a limited budget. Do, however, present yourself in proper attire.

Don't be late! If for some unavoidable reason you will be late, call ahead to let the interviewer know. When you arrive, explain why you were late, apologize, and settle in for your interview. If the employer cannot see you at a later time, ask if you can have a phone interview at a time that is convenient for the employer.

Salary Negotiations

The interviewer may ask you about salary requirements or expectations. Often this is done indirectly, by asking your salary history.

As a newly licensed pharmacist, you will not have a salary history. The employer knows this and may tell you what the starting salary is. If the employer presses you for a salary figure, tell him or her that you honestly do not know what to suggest and ask about the position's salary range.

If you think you may be asked to propose an acceptable starting salary, another strategy is to find out in advance what the company customarily offers someone with your background and experience.

Remember that base salary is not the only consideration. Ask about frequency of salary reviews and the basis for raises. For example, are cost-of-living raises routinely granted? Does the organization have a stepped-increase system based on length of service, or do raises depend on merit? Have wages been frozen in recent years?

Follow-up Letter

After the interview, write a thank-you letter. This is both a matter of courtesy and an opportunity to reiterate why you are the right person for the position. When there are several equally qualified applicants, the follow-up letter can be the determining factor. Make sure that you write down the names of everyone who interviewed you. Ask for business cards so that you can be sure of the correct spelling of each interviewer's name and title.

Making Your Decision

If you've done your research, created a top-notch résumé, and followed the other advice in this chapter, you're well on your way to a successful career search.

The offers will eventually come rolling in. As they do, a final word of advice. Don't be hasty. You don't have to accept the first offer you receive. At the same time, be sure that you don't aim too high at the beginning. Remember the words of Donna Walker-Pulido, one of the pharmacists profiled in Chapter 1: "You have to be willing to accept entry-level jobs to show your skills and to gain credibility within an organization or corporation. Build on experiences so that you can progress within the organization."

Job hunting can be a real balancing act. Keep in mind that pharmacy is a growth field. In most cases, the number of positions exceeds the supply of qualified pharmacists. Take your time, and have confidence in yourself.

Print Resources

Chain Pharmacy. The National Association of Chain Drug Stores (NACDS) publishes a membership directory in which you can find the name of the person to whom you should address employment inquiries. (This is usually the director of human resources or personnel.) NACDS sends the directory to pharmacy school deans each January. Check with your dean or contact the director of professional services at NACDS at (703) 549-3001.

Community Pharmacy. The *Hayes Directory* lists pharmacies in alphabetical order by state. Names of the owners or managers are not included. Be sure to call the pharmacy and get a contact name before sending a letter. The directory can be found at some college of pharmacy libraries.

For information, contact the publisher, Edward N. Hayes, 4229 Birch Street, Newport Beach, CA 92660; (714) 756-9063.

Hospital Pharmacy. Contact your state chapter of the American Society of Health-System Pharmacists (ASHP). Your dean's office will have this information.

ASHP also offers on-site career recruitment services at its Midyear Clinical and Annual Meetings, held in December and June, respectively. Students must submit application materials at least one month before the meeting. A message service is available for employers to contact applicants to schedule interviews on site.

For more information, contact ASHP's coordinator of student and resident affairs at ASHP at (301) 657-3000.

Federal Pharmacy. Federal Career Opportunities, a weekly publication, can help you find positions in the federal government. It is published by the Federal Research Service Inc., P.O. Box 1059, Vienna, VA 22180; (703) 281-0200.

Positions for pharmacists are available in many federal agencies, including the Public Health Service, Indian Health Service, National Institutes of Health, and Food and Drug Administration, as well as in the U.S armed forces.

To apply for a position in the federal government, you must be put on the national register. To do so, call your state's federal job information center and request a Pharmacists' Application Package. Your application will be evaluated and put on the register from which federal agencies recruit candidates. If selected, you will be contacted directly by the agency for an interview.

If you are interested in working for a Department of Veterans Affairs (VA) hospital, you must apply through the VA Special Examining Unit in addition to being listed on the federal register. Some of the armed services and other federal agencies use this service as well. For information and an application, call (800) 368-6008; in Virginia, call (800) 552-3045.

Many pharmaceutical manufacturers have Web pages that include position listings. A list of Web addresses appears at the end of this chapter. A quick browse of the Internet may yield some interesting career opportunities.

Other Resources

Both career planning centers at your college and university bookstores have books and guides on interviewing and résumé writing. Short courses are also available on these topics.

Two computer programs are available to help you write a résumé or vita. They are The Perfect Résumé and PFC: The Résumé Pro.

Books

Bolles RN. *What Color Is Your Parachute?* Ten Speed Press. Berkeley, CA. 1996.

Gable FB. *Opportunities in Pharmacy Careers.* National Textbook Company. 4255 W. Touhy Avenue, Lincolnwood, IL 60646. Hardback $9.95; paperback $6.95.

Rucker TD (ed). *Pharmacy: Career Planning and Professional Opportunities.* Health Administration Press. University of Michigan, 102 E. Horan Street, Ann Arbor, MI 48109. $24.

The Pfizer Guide: Pharmacy Career Opportunities. Merritt Communications Inc. 142 Ferry Road, Suite 13, Old Saybrook, CT 06475. Free.

Occupational Outlook Handbook. Bureau of Labor Statistics. Superintendent of Documents, U.S. Government Printing Office, Washington, DC 20402. Contains information on pharmacy employment opportunities. $8.50.

On-Line Resources

The following on-line resources are available to job hunters.

Begin all Web addresses with "http://".

Résumés

For a fee, you can post your résumé on the World Wide Web. Interested employers will contact you directly. The name of this service is A+ Online Résumés. Address: www.hway.com/olresume

AAA Résumé is a Web site that offers hints and services for job hunters. For a fee, the site will critique your résumé or write one for you. The site also has information about job searching and human resource issues. Address: www.infi.net/~resume/

Employment Listings

PharmWeek (www.pharminfo.com/pharmall). Weekly lists of openings in health-system pharmacy. If you send a photocopy of your pharmacy license, you will receive a free print copy of this list.

Jobs (www.cpb.uokhsc.edu/-pharmacy/jobs.html). List of pharmacy employment opportunities.

MedSearch America (www.medsearch.com). Employment opportunities in health.

RPh On-the-Go (interaccess.com/rph/Newjob.html).

Pharmaceutical Manufacturers

These sites contain career information as well as information on drug products and disease states.
- Abbott (www.abbott.com)
- Astra (www.astra.com)
- Bayer (www.bayer.com)
- Boehringer Ingelheim

- (www.boehringer-ingelheim.com)
- Bristol-Myers Squibb (www.bms.com)
- Ciba Geigy (www.ciba.com)
- Fischer (www.dr-fischer.com)
- Genentech (www.gene.com)
- Glaxo Wellcome (www.glaxowellcome.co.uk)
- Hoechst Marion Roussel (www.hoechst.com)
- Johnson & Johnson (www.jnj.com)
- Lilly (www.lilly.com)
- Merck (www.merck.com)
- Monsanto (www.monsanto.com)
- Mylan (www.mylan.com)
- Novartis (www.novartis.com)
- Novo Nordisk (www.novo.dkl)
- Pfizer (www.pfizer.com)
- Pharmacia & Upjohn (www.pnu.com)
- Rhone-Poulenc (www.calvacom.fr/rhonepoulenc)
- Roche (www.roche.com)
- Roxane (www.roxane.com)
- Schering-Plough (www.schering-pl.it)
- Searle (www.monsanto.com/searle)
- SmithKline Beecham (www.sb.com)
- Solvay (www.solvay.co)
- Taro (www.taropharma.com)
- 3M Pharmaceuticals (www.3m.com)
- Warner Lambert (www.warner-lambert.com)
- Zeneca (www.zeneca.com)

Appendix O

Sample Cover Letter

February 21, 1997

Joe Smith, Pharm.D.
Community Hospital
145 Forest Hill Road
Columbus, Ohio 43210

Dear Dr. Smith:

Thank you for taking the time to speak with me on the telephone the other day. It is always a pleasure to talk to someone "back home." As we discussed, I plan to return to Columbus after graduating with a B.S. degree in pharmacy from the University of Wisconsin in May. I will be taking the NAPLEX on June 28. I am very interested in working with you and your staff in the pharmacy at Community Hospital.

At the APhA-ASP Midyear Regional Meeting last November, I told you of my plans to do an externship at Good Samaritan Medical Center in Madison, Wisconsin. I have now completed nearly half of the externship and I am finding the experience very rewarding. I realize now that I would like to pursue a career in hospital pharmacy. When I complete the externship at Good Samaritan, I will have worked in the central pharmacy and in three satellite pharmacies—surgery, pediatrics, and oncology. My experiences as a pharmacy extern have taught me about the many services hospital pharmacists can offer, from patient counseling to nutritional assessment and inservice training courses for nurses and other health professionals.

I respect the quality services that Community Hospital offers and would like to put my knowledge and experience to use in such a fine practice. I believe that my leadership skills developed while serving as vice president of the University of Wisconsin's chapter of the APhA Academy of Students of Pharmacy also will translate into usable management skills.

My résumé is enclosed for your review. I hope we can talk soon about the opportunities available at Community Hospital. I will be home for spring break between March 12 and 20, and will call you on March 14 to set up a visit. If you wish to call me, my number is (608) 262-3434 on campus and (614) 422-6781 at home in Columbus.

Sincerely,

Mary Jones
1220 University Drive
Madison, WI 53706

Appendix P

Sample Résumé

MARY JONES

School Address:
1220 University Drive
Madison, WI 53706
(608) 262-3434

Permanent Address:
10 Shady Lane
Columbus, OH 43210
(614) 422-6781

Career Objective: To pursue a career as a hospital pharmacist

Education: University of Wisconsin School of Pharmacy:
B.S. in Pharmacy, 1998

Experience: Pharmacy Externships

1994-97 — Pharmacy Extern, Towne Pharmacy, Madison, WI. Performed dispensing functions. Counseled patients on prescription and nonprescription medications. Helped design software for personalized patient information. Initiated and promoted a weekly blood pressure monitoring service, which gave the pharmacy greater visibility and helped bring in new patients.

1/97 to 3/97 — Pharmacy Extern, Good Samaritan Medical Center, Madison, WI. Helped prepare unit-dose distribution and IV admixture in the central pharmacy and in surgery, pediatrics, and oncology satellite pharmacies. Initiated contact with discharge planning team and worked with them to start involving the pharmacy department in medication counseling for patients being discharged. Participated in medical rounds, assisted with nutritional assessment, made recommendations to physicians regarding composition of hyperalimentation formulae, and helped prepare hyperalimentation solutions. Designed and presented inservice training course for nurses comparing the third-generation cephalosporins.

Professional Activities: American Pharmaceutical Association Academy of Students of Pharmacy, 1993 to present
- Chapter vice president, 1996-97. Planned and oversaw all professional activities, including blood glucose monitoring and Medic Alert program and fund raising, which increased the chapter's treasury by 25% from previous year.
- Chairman of Community Hypertension Screening Committee, 1995-96. Organized and directed daylong hypertension screening service in shopping mall, which served over 100 people. Planned and set up "Hypertension Month" display at a local hospital. Wrote an article for the state pharmacy association journal about the chapter's hypertension activities.
- Health editor of university newspaper, 1995-97. Wrote four columns a year on health topics such as cough and cold preparations, acne medications, sunburn remedies, and topical steroids.
- Gave presentation on drug abuse to seventh grade class at local junior high.

Honors: Who's Who Among American Colleges and Universities, 1996
Rho Chi Honor Society, 1996 to present
Phi Lambda Sigma Leadership Society, 1996 to present
APhA-ASP Mortar and Pestle Professionalism Award, 1988

Appendix Q

Sample Curriculum Vitae

David L. Hammersmith, Pharm.D.
1902 N. Noonan Street
Irvington, VA 23201
(804) 999-9999
E-mail: dlhamm@aol.com

EDUCATION

1983-87 Doctor of Pharmacy, College of Pharmacy, University of Minnesota, Minneapolis
1980-83 Premedicine/Prepharmacy Studies, College of Liberal Arts
University of Minnesota, Minneapolis

PROFESSIONAL EXPERIENCE

9/93-9/96	Clinical Coordinator, Critical Care and Transplantation, Department of Pharmacy Services; The Medical Center
3/92-9/93	Assistant Director of Pharmacy Services; The Medical Center
1987-3/92	Clinical Pharmacist, East Nebraska Hospital; Affiliate Assistant Professor of Pharmacy Practice, Creighton University School of Pharmacy

PROFESSIONAL LICENSURE AND CERTIFICATION

1992	Virginia by reciprocity
1991	Board Certified in Pharmacotherapy
1989	Advanced Cardiac Life Support—Instructor

PROFESSIONAL MEMBERSHIPS

Society of Critical Care Medicine
Virginia Pharmaceutical Association
American Pharmaceutical Association
Minnesota Pharmacy Alumni Association

SPEAKERS' BUREAUS

Merck, Sharp and Dohme
Hoechst Marion Roussel Pharmaceuticals

HONORS AND AWARDS

1992	Who's Who in the Midwest
1992	Distinguished Young Pharmacist

RECENT JOB DESCRIPTION

From 1993 until 1996, I was Clinical Coordinator of Pharmacy Services at The Medical Center (TMC). TMC is a 650-bed community hospital with many tertiary services. In the capacity of clinical coordinator, I managed two satellite pharmacies (critical care and operating room); provided patient-centered care to 36 intensive-care-unit beds (medicine, surgery/trauma, cardiovascular) and solid organ transplant patients. I served on many interdisciplinary committees and process management teams.

PUBLICATIONS/POSTERS

Hammersmith DL. Fine-tuning a formulary. DICP, Ann Pharmacother. 1990 (April):H-1 to H-20.
Parker CM, Hammersmith DL. An old scourge: Tuberculosis in the 1990's. US Pharm. 1994;16(10):37-82.

POSTERS

Reduction in Unintentional Extubations among Agitated ICU Patients: An Algorithm for Sedation. Windom P, Warder B, Hammersmith DL, Roman MP, Traskil AT, Rainer TS. SCCM Annual Meeting and Exposition, February 1996.

PROFESSIONAL AND PUBLIC LECTURES
GENERAL:

1993-95	ACLS teaching four times/year; community education in transplantation three times/year; community and health professional education monthly

INVITED:

10/96	Understanding Homeopathy: Is It Really an Alternative to Medicine? Medical Transcriptionists Annual Meeting.
11/95	Inotropes and Vasodilators. AACN Fall Meeting.
5/95	The Effect of ICU Antibiotics on Resistance, panel presentation and discussion. AACN NTI.
4/95	Current Strategies in Balancing Neuromuscular Blockade and Sedation in the Intensive Care Unit. First Annual Advances in Pulmonary Diseases Conference.

APPOINTMENTS, COMMITTEES, AND OFFICES HELD

1997-	Editorial Board, *American Journal of Health-System Pharmacy*
1995-	American Pharmaceutical Association: Guidebook on Disease-Specific Pharmaceutical Care Protocols Member, Infectious Disease Panel
1990-	Society of Critical Care Medicine Member, Quality Indicator Committee

PROGRAM DEVELOPMENT

1994:
Developer of a Critical Care/Nutrition Support Specialty Residency. One resident completed program in 1994-95.

"Hospital Pharmacy Practice Update." September 13, 1991. Invitational continuing-education program directed at hospital pharmacists. Support from Merck, Sharp and Dohme ($4,000).

Second Annual "Spring Research and Practice Conference." May 3, 1991. Invitational conference for Nebraska pharmacy leaders and pharmacy faculty. Support from Merck, Sharp and Dohme, The Upjohn Company, and Hoechst Roussel ($2,850).

Notes

Notes

Notes

Notes

Notes

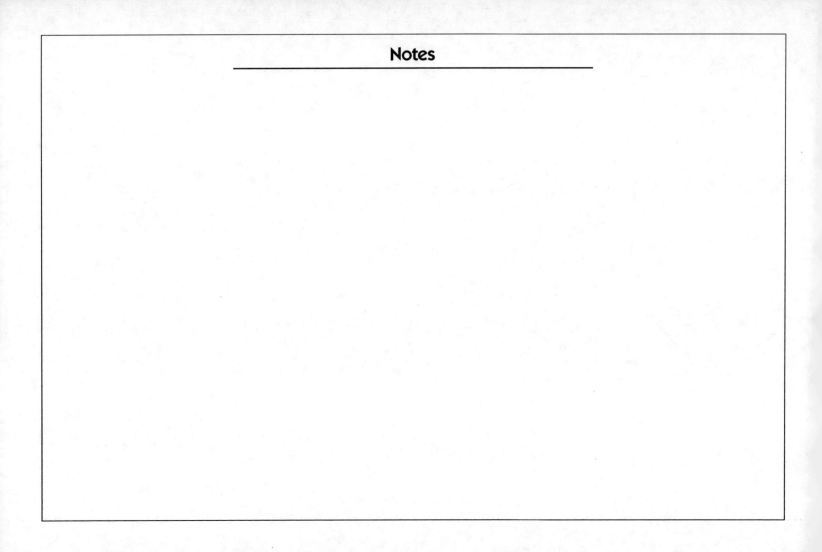

Notes

Notes